Nursing Centers:
The Time Is Now

Nursing Centers: The Time Is Now

Barbara Murphy
Editor

National League for Nursing Press • New York
Pub. No. 41-2629

ISBN 0-88737-623-1

This book was set in Palatino by Publications Development Company. The designer was Allan Graubard. The editor was Maryan Malone. The cover was designed by Lauren Stevens.

Printed in the United States of America

Contents

CONTENTS

Contributors

Jeanette Adams, DrPH, RN, University of Texas-Houston, Houston, TX

Kimberly Adams-Davis, MSN, RN C, OGNP, Frances Payne Bolton School of Nursing, Case Western Reserve University, Cleveland, OH

Janice S. Borman, PhD, RN, Saint Xavier University, Chicago IL

Norman D. Brown, EdD, RN, University of Arkansas for Medical Sciences, College for Nursing, Little Rock, AR

Nancy Chevalier, MS, RN, PNP, University of Rochester School of Nursing, Rochester, NY

Peter Coggiola, MSN, RN C, University of Rochester School of Nursing, Rochester, NY

Colleen M. Dwyer, MS, RN, NP C, University of Rochester School of Nursing, Rochester, NY

Lorna Finnegan, MS, RN, Saint Xavier University, Chicago IL

Joyce J. Fitzpatrick, PhD, RN, FAAN, Frances Payne Bolton School of Nursing, Case Western Reserve University, Cleveland, OH

Sue Groth, MS, RN, NP C, University of Rochester School of Nursing, Rochester, NY

Donna Hill, PhD, RN, NP C, University of Rochester School of Nursing, Rochester, NY

Carol Ann Lockhart, PhD, RN, FAAN, C. Lockhart Associates, Tempe, AZ

Sally Peck Lundeen, PhD, RN, FAAN, University of Wisconsin–Milwaukee, Milwaukee, WI

Thomas Mackey, PhD, RN C, University of Texas-Houston, Houston, TX

Terri L. Mileham, MS, RN, FNP, Arizona State University College of Nursing, Tempe, AZ

Linda Moneyham, DNS, RN, Nell Hodgson Woodruff School of Nursing, Emory University, Atlanta, GA

Barbara Murphy, EdD, RN, National League for Nursing, New York, NY

Ruth M. Neil, PhD, RN, University of Colorado School of Nursing, Denver, CO

Mary Oesterle, EdD, RN, Saint Xavier University, Chicago IL

Phyllis J. Primas, PhD, RN, Arizona State University College of Nursing, Tempe, AZ

Lenoa Michelle Rios, MS, RN C, FNP, UCLA School of Nursing Health Center, Los Angeles, CA

Cecelia B. Scott, Programs Assisting Community Elderly, Inc., Roswell, GA

Adrienne Springer, MS, RN, PNP, University of Rochester School of Nursing, Rochester, NY

Anthony Suchman, MD, Highland Hospital, Rochester, NY

Susan Swider, PhD, RN, Saint Xavier University, Chicago IL

Mary Jane Tranzillo, MSN, RN, University of Medicine and Dentistry of New Jersey School of Nursing, Newark, NJ

John M. Walker, MA, University of Rochester School of Nursing, Rochester, NY

Patricia Hinton Walker, PhD, RN, FAAN, University of Rochester School of Nursing, Rochester, NY

Preface

The year 1994 will go down in the annals of history as a year of intense debate on major national health care reform and as "the year the music died" in Congress once again on that important issue. Regardless of any future outcome at the national level, however, the debate has afforded numerous opportunities for professional nursing, in general, and those of us invested in the evolution of nursing centers, in particular, to speak out. We have used these opportunities to move ahead a much needed agenda for change. It is at the local and state levels that this impetus for change must be kept alive across the country for it is at the local level that the seeds of lasting change are nurtured.

Nursing centers provide individuals direct access to services based on nursing models of care. Although nurses are essential providers of clinical services in almost all health care delivery settings, consumers do not always have direct access to these nurses, nor are many delivery systems based on nursing models of care. Nursing centers provide an opportunity for consumers to have direct access to nurses who have developed innovative, nontraditional prevention and intervention strategies and models of health care delivery.

These models vary widely from one another, supporting the emphasis on consumer-focused care that is another basic element of the working definition of "nursing center" as refined by the National League for Nursing Council on Nursing Centers. It is a great strength of the nursing center movement that multiple nursing center models are being developed, implemented, and modified across the country in response to specific community needs and the active participation and feedback of consumers. This dynamic, consumer-focused change process is the very hallmark of creative, local health policy reform.

Nursing centers also have the unique potential of providing the cornerstone for health care reform by facilitating the development of collaborative models of health and health care delivery. Collaborative models acknowledge that no single professional discipline is able to provide the array of programs and services necessary to meet the health and health-related needs of individuals, families, and communities. Nurses, physicians, social workers, dentist, psychologists, holistic healers, allied health professionals, nutritionists, and others bring both expertise and unique perspectives to the cure and/or care of illness, and the maintenance of health. Collaborative models will result in practice that focuses on the broader vision of enabling each of us to constantly strive for improved health status as well as gain easy access to the treatments for disrupted health when necessary.

Collaborative models will result in professionals and paraprofessionals in the area of education, recreation, employment, day care, religion, and others joining health providers in an attempt to coordinate programs and reduce fragmentation of service delivery. Collaborative models will embrace consumers as active partners in the assessment of need, development of intervention strategies, and evaluation of services. In short, the future of successful reform will rest on the ability of professionals from various disciplines to collaborate with each other and consumers to develop health oriented models of service delivery.

Professional nurses understand the strengths and weaknesses of both medical care and health care models. Professional nurses understand the need to develop models to meet the health needs of the entire community as well as those of individuals and families. For decades, many advanced practice nurses and community health nurses have had to be knowledgeable about and proficient in medical, mental health, and public health interventions. Nursing centers have the unique opportunity to define and facilitate the development of much stronger links between the existing public health and medical service delivery systems and between health providers and systems of all types and other human service providers and systems. This is the real challenge for future health policy reform.

Nurses must continue to define and describe the elements of unique nursing center practice that are unique and those that are similar to other settings. We must modify and expand our nursing roles in relation to consumer needs and other disciplines. Nurses do have a unique contribution to make, but we can't do it alone. We must demonstrate the vision and wisdom necessary to effectively collaborate with colleagues and consumers and to provide role models of innovative collaboration for others to follow. It is an exciting and challenging time to be a part of the growing cadre of colleagues involved in nursing center development and research. With creativity and perseverance, nursing centers can lead the way by example to an era of true health policy reform.

Sally Peck Lundeen, PhD, RN, FAAN
Chair, NLN Council for Nursing Centers

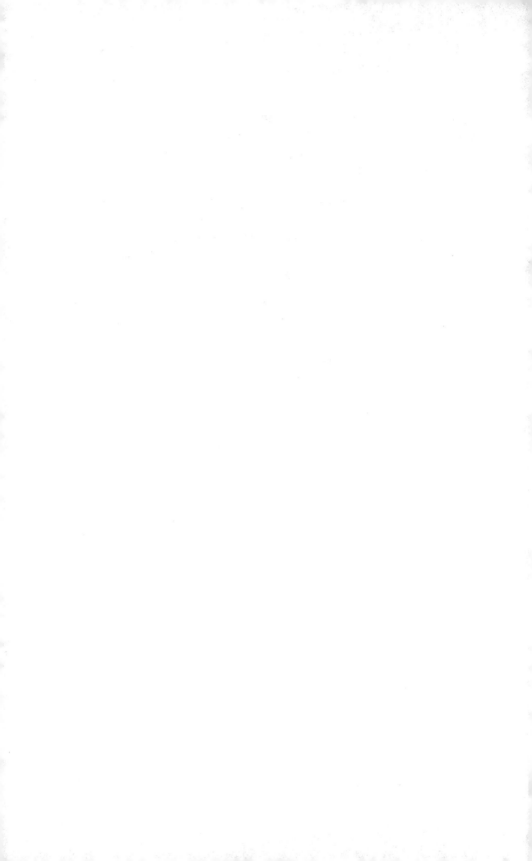

Introduction

A brief history of the nursing centers movement will provide readers with the background information to appreciate the movement's roots, evolution, and hope for the future. Issues of the past resurface in the present. Feelings of connectedness with those who helped bring us to this point will also help to guide our futures.

Nursing centers, owned and or operated by nurses who promote health and provide nursing services directly to clients, trace their origin to the Henry Street Settlement founded by Lillian Wald in 1893. Through this organization the sick and impoverished of New York City were provided with health teaching and nursing care. In 1965, the establishment of the nurse practitioner role, in which nurses provide primary nursing care to clients, manage and monitor their health needs, and make appropriate referrals, heralded the beginning of nursing centers as they are known today. The 1970s marked the beginning of many university based or academic nursing centers which were established to provide community services, learning experiences for students, and settings for faculty practice and research. In 1978, O. Marie Henry, in her address to the American Public Health Association, charged nurses to develop new means for providing nursing care and delivering nursing services. She urged nurses to establish nursing centers in institutional, community, and primary care settings. In response to this charge, the 1980s saw a proliferation of many types of nursing centers: academic based, hospital based, and free standing nurse-managed agencies for home health care.

In May 1982, at the first national conference on nursing centers, nurses met collectively to share their experiences and to find support thereby. In 1984, at their second national conference, the group formulated a definition of nursing centers that encompassed the provision of holistic, client-centered health services using a nursing model. Health promotion, disease prevention, and collaboration with other health care professionals were identified as integral components of the mission of nursing centers. Along with providing health services directly to clients, many of the centers also had as part of their purpose the provision of a site for student learning, faculty practice, and research. In 1986, at the group's third national conference, participants identified the need to become a part of a national organization to further promote their mission and goals in a more formalized and global manner. In 1988, this lead to the integration of the nursing centers group into the membership of the National League for Nursing and the formation of a special interest council within the League named the Council for Nursing Centers (CNC).

As an integral part of the National League for Nursing, the Council for Nursing Centers has continued to promote its mission through a variety of educational programs, publications, research initiatives, and ad hoc committee work. Members of the Council have mentored and provided consultation to their colleagues in support of advancing the concept of nursing centers as affordable, quality, and accessible alternatives to our present health care delivery system.

In keeping with the Council's mission, this publication is being offered to those many nurses, other health care providers, and community members who have been seeking to learn more about this growing movement. The contributors to this publication are all members of the NLN Council for Nursing Centers. In their writings you will find true creativity mingled with the drive and the spirit that has always been a hallmark of nurses who chose to be involved in nursing centers.

This publication is divided into three sections. The first section is comprised of five chapters that deal with subject matter in a more global manner; information and issues that have broad application to all nursing centers.

The first chapter offers an analysis of community nursing centers based on a study conducted for the Robert Wood Johnson Foundation. The descriptive information presented relative to nursing centers around the country, their strengths, weaknesses, and issues of survival provide a helpful background to subsequent chapters. This information is based on a review of the literature, an analysis of other surveys conducted on nursing centers, phone interviews, and site visits. The findings of this study point up the wide variations in nursing centers' models as well as services provided. Findings will be reinforced in later chapters devoted to showcasing specific centers.

Issues raised and discussed in Chapter 1 include: financing and reimbursement for services; roadblocks to practice, including competition with physicians; marketing and business strategies; and legal concerns including licensing and liability.

The chapter concludes with a list of ten observations about the challenges that will need to be addressed for advanced practice nurses to be fairly positioned at the healthcare reform table. The findings of this study will be validated over and over again in subsequent chapters of this book.

Chapter 2 opens with a discussion of the Health Security Act (HSA), now of historic value in that it succeeded in propelling health care reform to the forefront of the Clinton Administration's domestic policy considerations and in so doing forced Americans at all levels to become more acutely aware of the complex issues surrounding health care reform and to engage them in meaningful dialogue with policy makers. As these debates continue to mold and shape the future of health care delivery in the United States, the Clinton HSA will be viewed as a true benchmark.

The real strength of this chapter, however, lies in the author's discussion of the opportunities the healthcare reform debate has created for advanced practice nurses (APNs) to educate the uninformed regarding nurses' unique roles as primary care providers prepared to address issues of cost containment, comprehensive systems of care, and preparation of a diverse health professions work force. The author offers a wealth of suggestions regarding what nurses can do to position themselves as pivotal in this changing health care environment. He also explores a wide variety of complex issues such as development of collaborative models of practice between physicians and nurses in the integrated delivery systems of the future.

Outcomes-oriented research, culturally sensitive care, supply and demand, insurance reform, expanded practice acts are other areas explored. Throughout his discussions the author makes the case for why APNs and nursing centers are the solution to accessible, quality, cost-effective and consumer-oriented care.

Chapter 3 focuses on the value and demonstrated success of basing a nursing center on nursing theory, in this case, Watson's philosophy and science of human caring. The author makes a strong case for how this theory provides the cohesiveness around which the nursing care of HIV/AIDS clients is practiced. The key message here is that nursing, as a practice discipline, has a responsibility not only to provide care of the utmost quality but to base that care on a body of knowledge generated through "reflective practice and scientific inquiry." The author makes a strong case for how nursing centers provide the ideal setting for refining and enhancing the unique contributions nurses bring to the health care delivery arena.

The nursing center's mission statement, which "articulates shared beliefs and values and provides guidance for all center decisions," along with the seven major assumptions of Watson's theory are presented and discussed. To reinforce the success of this model, practice outcomes such as steady growth, cost savings to sponsoring agencies, and client/staff satisfaction are identified.

The next two chapters focus on management information systems (MIS) in community nursing centers (CNCs). In the first of these two chapters, Chapter 4, the author presents an overview of the many reasons why accurate and appropriate data collection is so critical. Emphasis is placed on the importance of outcomes data to the long-term viability of CNCs. Also emphasized is the role of relational data bases in producing answers to complex questions such as the nature of reimbursement policies and practices as they relate to primary prevention as a nursing intervention.

Organizations that lack a planned strategy as well as methods and procedures for obtaining and using appropriate information technology will end up with fragmented and incompatible communications as well as insufficient service delivery. Chapter 5 offers a step-by-step narrative of how to develop and implement a strategic plan for a comprehensive information system in a nursing center and is richly supplemented with charts and resources. These expert authors carefully describe how to analyze the business functions of a center and the processes and activities to identify both present and future information needs to support these functions. Tips about pitfalls to avoid, such as choosing a system that is incapable of a longitudinal analysis of selected variables when a history of change is required, are also shared. Another key contribution is a discussion of the criteria for selection of software packages and the pros and cons of off-the-shelf vs. design-your-own packages. Additional practical tips such as information about software integration, the software package's capabilities to export and import data from and to other specialized software packages, make this a must read.

Chapters 6 through 12 are devoted to showcasing specific nursing centers models and, in so doing, to demonstrate their individual uniqueness. Specific examples show how advanced practice nurses are in tune with the needs of their communities, are responsive to these needs, provide culturally sensitive health care services, and are quick to respond in creative, visionary, and even tenacious ways. Successes are related to building community support in true collaborative models.

In Chapter 6, the authors describe a series of circumstances that lead them from one very specific event, the closure of a health care facility, to an in-depth community assessment revealing a broad range of community health care needs and the building of strong public/private support that helped defray many of the start-up costs of the center.

A unique feature of this chapter is the candid discussion of the many obstacles confronted by the authors (most of which were of a state regulatory nature) and how they were overcome. In their discussions of their experiences around such issues as passage of state legislation granting pilot demonstration status to their center, the authors show how many of the suggestions made previously in Chapter 2 can be operationalized.

Chapter 7 describes the establishment of a partnership between an urban university school of nursing and a public elementary school located in a medically underserved community. This partnership resulted in the establishment of a consumer-driven, community-based nursing center providing family centered primary health care. The activities of the center in its first seven months including community assessment and collaboration, delivery of services, and the evaluation of quality cost-effectiveness outcomes are described.

An important contribution here is a discussion of the training and utilization of community health advocates (CHAs). The CHA, a community resident and bridge to the community and the health system, helps to bring services to the community and to mobilizes residents to improve their health and living conditions. A helpful description of the activities of the CHA and the CHA training program are detailed.

The evolution of an autonomous innovative rural practice developed through a university community nursing center is the focal point of Chapter 8. The author, a nurse practitioner, addresses access, cost effectiveness, and quality in care delivery to underserved populations, emphasizing the entrepreneurial and intrepreneurial skills needed to achieve these goals. The faculty practice described here consists of three sites: the county jail, where holistic primary health care services are provided to the inmates; a family health care center (owned by a community hospital) where family care is provided in the community including care to homebound patients; and a mobile health unit (converted from a 38-foot recreational vehicle) providing community primary care in front of the local fire house.

Highlights of this chapter include: a chronology of the development of each component of the practice addressing overcoming obstacles; contract development to generate sufficient revenue to support the practice; and the use of case study examples to demonstrate the value and effectiveness of the NP faculty practice role in rural settings.

In the present-day health care reform climate where integrated delivery systems, managed care, and interdisciplinary approaches to delivery of services are being explored, Chapter 9 is especially timely. The author focuses on the development of a collaborative practice between physicians and nurse practitioners (NPs) from: how it all began, to the overcoming of obstacles, to plans for its future. This chapter provides a clear, detailed description of the development of a true collaborative practice where NP and MD work in partnership rather than where the NP works in subordination to the MD. The many factors that contribute to the success of this collaboration are discussed, not the least of which is the establishment of equality through comparable faculty ranking and reciprocal consultations.

This chapter is enriched by case study examples which emphasize the critical contributions of advanced practice nurses using a holistic care approach as described in the Neuman Systems Model. An added plus is the case made for the use of marketing to educate about the role of the NP, what services the NP can provide that are uniquely nursing, and what the benefits of a collaborative practice are over using a single provider.

Because adolescent health care has challenged providers for decades, Chapter 10 is an especially important resource for those seeking successful outcomes in this extremely vulnerable population. In her descriptions of the needs of this population, enhanced through the use of specific cased study examples, the author's sensitivity and clinical expertise are clearly demonstrated.

Creative new practice models of care using advanced practice nurses are described. Specific activities that have been identified as responsible for positive outcomes include: providing services to adolescents on their own turf, in school based clinics, group home settings, neighborhood health clinics, sports camps, churches, recreation/community settings, shelters; employing a flex-firm approach of collaboration among practitioners, in this case the school nurse practitioner, pediatric nurse practitioner, and women's health practitioner; working with other agencies and providers to fill gaps in provision of services; providing client centered services delivered in both an age-sensitive and culture-sensitive manner; and creative problem solving such as job sharing to address the challenges of rural health care delivery. The important message skillfully reinforced throughout this chapter is the special strengths of the nurse practitioner in the delivery of care that is reliable, responsive, continuing, and caring.

The nursing profession's strength in identifying gaps in the provision of health care services and in finding creative ways to fill those gaps is clearly reinforced by the example presented in Chapter 11. Services provided to children of the working poor who are not eligible to be insured by the Arizona Health Care Cost Containment System (the state's managed care program for medicaid eligible clients) are detailed. Three interacting dimensions: aggressive community outreach, portable clinics which deliver primary care organized by stations through which clients move to receive various aspects of services, and a comprehensive referral and follow-up system are detailed.

The important contributions of this chapter are many. The description of a true collaborative model which engages an advisory board made up of state and local community groups suggests the use of a combination of resources not frequently identified in the literature. An extensive and comprehensive assessment of primary care needs, supplementing the use of a community advisory board with the use of computer mapping to determine geographic areas of priority is also presented. How to begin and how to evolve through the development of an "entire mini-health care system" from personnel recruitment, to creative staffing patterns using only part-time professional staff complemented by extensive use of volunteers, to policy and procedure development, to the establishment of computerized record keeping, to aggressive marketing enrich the contributions of these authors.

Chapter 12 describes the formation of a student health center established in response to the school of nursing's need to monitor compliance with the university's health and immunization policy. The center idea was marketed to other schools within the university as a solution to the problems they were also experiencing regarding lost records and fragmented follow-up services.

A collaborative model is described whereby the school of nursing worked with the information systems and technology department to develop computerized record keeping and reporting systems. From these beginnings has evolved the concept of the development of a health assessment center where students could not only meet the requirements of the university's student health policies but also receive affordable health care provided by nurse practitioners. Featured here is the author's description of the responsibilities and activities of the center's administrator along with an analysis of the outcomes of the services provided to students. Also helpful to the reader is a discussion of future plans including a candid discussion of the issues/obstacles that the author feels will need to be overcome. Finally, the formation of a professional corporation among the school of nursing, university mental health services, and health related services is described relative to the potential this collaboration holds for the provision of a wider range of services to the student and the community.

The final chapters of this book focus on research studies conducted by advance practice nurses in their centers. The keen assessment and analytical skills of these nurse researchers as well as their connectedness to the populations they serve is a powerful testament to the importance of their contributions to the health of our communities.

The underlying message of Chapter 13, is a plea to nurses to conduct research studies in nursing centers which address four key areas: consumer needs not met in our present system, nursing interventions designed to address those needs, the achievement of positive outcomes, and the demonstration of cost-effectiveness of services provided by nurses. The authors/ researchers present data from a recent phenomenological study which they conducted that incorporated a focus group methodology. The purpose of the study was to examine the perceptions and experiences of older adults using the services of an on-site community-based nursing center. The study identified autonomous nursing interventions valued by consumers as well as concomitant outcomes related to health. Data generated from the study indicated that services deemed as necessary or desirable to the enhancement of the subjects sense of health and well-being extended beyond the traditional physical illness-oriented care provided by the physician. Access to care, psychosocial interventions, and environmental issues were among the many needs being addressed in the nursing center. Through the sharing of conversations with clients, enriched by many specific quotes, the authors are able to document the many essential services that nurses are able to provide that are not being provided by any other caregiver.

If ever the case was made for the importance of culturally sensitive health care delivery, it is made in this next chapter, Chapter 14. The author skillfully describes a special situation in which her unique combination of skills as a bilingual pediatric nurse practitioner led to positive client outcomes as well as a significant contribution to the body of nursing knowledge on patterns of psychomotor and language development in Hispanic immigrant/poor children. The author's assessment skills are combined with her ability to question patterns of development in a qualitative research environment and to validate emerging patterns through an extensive review of the literature which included not only nursing but extended to the disciplines of education and psychology as well. Her ability to draw on her theoretical knowledge base along with her clinical practice and personal multicultural experiences provided valuable tools to compare and contrast the developmental patterns of these Hispanic children to other populations. One of the key factors leading to the selection of interventions that achieved positive outcomes was the uncovering of bilingual communication practices that explained response behaviors, accomplished through the author's ability to understand the culture of the Hispanic immigrant/poor coupled with her fluency in both English and Spanish.

The final chapter of this book, Chapter 15, describes one aspect of a program of health promotion conducted through a nursing center. The use of a self-administered health risk appraisal questionnaire is described as well as the research study conducted to determine the value of such an instrument in assessing employee health status at a large health science university. Detailed information is provided regarding considerations to be addressed in choosing an appropriate health appraisal instrument in the areas of: validity, reliability, and population sampling. A candid discussion of the results of a cost/benefits analysis, the significance of health related outcomes to both clients and providers and implications for the future are also highlights of this chapter.

By sharing their experiences and their stories, the contributors of this book have succeeded in defining themselves. They have answered two questions: what is a nursing center and what are the roles of advanced practice nurses in these settings? Though there are wide variations in the populations served, the services provided, and the ways in which these services are delivered, a clear and unifying message is consistent throughout each chapter. Advanced practice nurses in nursing centers today are more like than unlike Lillian Wald and her Henry Street Settlement. They know, as she did, that change occurs outside the system not within it; that change requires a lot of perseverance, creativity, and hard work; and that the answer to meeting our health care crisis lies within a community-based nursing model focused on health promotion, disease prevention, and interdisciplinary collaboration. Most of all, nurses in nursing centers know that health care delivery is a partnership endeavor, a partnership of working *with* clients, not *for* clients, a partnership of working *with* communities, not *in* communities. Thank you all for sending that message so clearly.

Barbara Murphy, EdD, RN
Vice President for Council Affairs and
Director, Council for Nursing Centers

1

Community Nursing Centers: An Analysis of Status and Needs

Carol Ann Lockhart

Never lose your idealism
Tip O'Neill, 1994

CAROL ANN LOCKHART

STRUCTURE AND METHODOLOGY OF THE ANALYSIS

In this chapter, I present an analysis of the current state of Community Nursing Centers (CNCs). The analysis is part of a larger effort of the Robert Wood Johnson Foundation, to keep abreast of developments specific to the U.S. health care system.

What is the current status of Community Nursing Centers and why do some thrive while others fail? In addressing these questions, I turned to relevant financing, regulatory, and public policy issues, including: (1) a review of the literature; (2) an analysis of existing surveys of CNCs; and (3) semi-structured telephone interviews and site visits in 18 states with 40 individuals informed about and involved with the creation, development, and support of nursing centers of various size and type. Interviewed as well were representatives of relevant associations to determine issues of concern to their members.

The interviews and resource materials suggest a surprisingly consistent set of themes and issues that Community Nursing Centers face nationwide. Although not a random sample, those interviewed represent a geographically and programmatically diverse group of people and centers. The same problems and questions were raised by them so frequently that the observations and conclusions discussed below seem to represent a responsible assessment of the viability of, and areas of need among, CNCs.

Definition of Community Nursing Centers

The term *Community Nursing Centers* was used in this study because of the presumed familiarity interviewees would have with it. It is used by the largest organized association of centers, the National League for Nursing's Council for Nursing Centers (established in 1988), and it was used in the NLN's 1991 survey

This chapter is prepared with the permission of the Robert Wood Johnson Foundation.

of the nearly 250 centers it identified. Phrases such as *nursing center, nurse-managed center, community nursing center, nurse-run clinic,* and *community nursing organization,* however, are all used interchangeably (Aydelotte et al., 1987; Riesch, 1992).

The NLN defines a Community Nursing Center as one where: (1) a nurse occupies the chief management position; (2) accountability and responsibility for client care and professional practice remains with nursing staff; and (3) nurses are the primary providers seen by clients visiting the center.

Interviewees stressed that a nursing center, however, is not only as a setting where clients visit, but also a concept which shapes the broader services offered by nurses in practice arrangements in the community (Aydelotte et al., 1987; Sharp, 1992; Riesch, 1990). There was general agreement that the definition of a CNC must encompass more than just one or several sites of care. It must allow for an actual site for care but also support nurse-managed services to clients in their home, community, hospital, nursing home or any site across the health care continuum.

The current brochure form the University of Rochester's Community Nursing Center reflects this thinking. It describes CNCs as, ". . . organizations which enable clients to contract directly with professional nurses for health care services rendered in community settings."

Types of Centers

The history of the development of CNCs will not be discussed here. However, a discussion of the types of centers which exist is necessary to explain how interviewees were chosen.

Susan Riesch (1992) categorizes nursing centers as: **community outreach**—free-standing centers similar to traditional community public health clinics; **institution-based**—which derive their mission from a large parent organization (hospital, university, corporation); and **wellness/health-promotion models**—to provide triage, screening, education, counseling, and health maintenance services. A fourth, loosely defined category has been described by Aydelotte et al. (1988) as **independent practice nurses** (faculty, nurse entrepreneurs).

In selecting centers for interview, we attempted to draw a sampling with differing affiliations, organizational relationships, and specialty areas. We interviewed people at: (1) community clinics (public or nonprofit free-standing); (2) institutionally related centers (academic, hospital and HMO (health maintenance organization); and (3) private nursing practices (entrepreneurs).

The Riesch distinction of a wellness/health promotion model was not useful since it did not distinguish between centers. Today, many centers have a wellness component, and although a number of academic centers began with this as a focus, most are now offering primary care, wellness, and other services. Other institutionally related categories or private arrangements might also be appropriate but are not prevalent at this time.

Last, although we used the word *entrepreneurial* to describe the private nursing practice, this does not mean some of the centers we encountered in other categories were not decidedly entrepreneurial.

FINDINGS

CNC Services

Community nursing centers offer a mix of medical acute care/ illness management and nursing care, coordination, and education services. Two almost parallel streams of service are offered. In one, advanced practice nurses (ANPs) offer medically-oriented care which seeks to be reimbursable under various insurance mechanisms. In the second, community health and other nurses provide a range of nursing care, coordination, and education which is not usually reimbursable under insurance plans but may be paid for through grants or contracts.

The CNC people we spoke with stressed a nursing philosophy of care and caring. They believe it is this philosophy which sets the community nursing centers apart from other centers that focus on medical cure. Even though nursing centers must strive to generate revenue under a largely medical care model, they want to be sure they do not lose sight of the approach which gives them the basis for their existence. Several expressed concern that financial pressures are already causing some to lose sight of that focus.

Another concern expressed was the isolationist nature of some nursing centers. Even though there is a different philosophy or approach, people stressed the need to build cooperative relationships with the community members themselves and other local providers. If the centers hope to survive, they must be part of the community and have good working relationships with physicians, pharmacists, and others who might serve their clients. As one CNC staff person said, "They must be embedded in the community."

Payment for Services

A number of centers reported a reluctance among nurses running CNCs to charge clients for care, even when to do so means the clinic may not survive. Several others said they had no need to learn about payment practices because of proposed national health care reform initiatives. They suggested the move to some prepaid system would negate any worry they might have about the payment process since it would no longer be relevant.

Contrasted with these attitudes are those expressed by center staff members who are cognizant of or actually manage multiple sources of revenue and a broad base of normally billed services. Here, payment practices and reimbursement, in general, are a matter of concern. In these centers, viability does seem more assured. Simply, they have worked around limitations on payment or practice. Some centers have gone directly to an employer or local and state governments for contracts. Others have convinced hospitals faced with high costs that they can reduce their costs with the use of a nursing center. Still others have negotiated payments from HMOs by showing them the impact they have on patient care problems and the costs avoided. A few have created a corporation so the insurer pays the corporation (as do many when they pay a hospital) rather than individuals, thereby sidestepping questions about of "who" gets paid.

Even with these successes, access to payment for all types of medical and nursing services remains the necessary element if CNCs are to survive. Restrictions on the payment and practice of Advanced Nurse Practitioners (ANPs) was overwhelmingly identified as one of the most limiting factors in the long-term viability of centers. Even so, the headaches involved in getting access to payments are more than some centers believe the return is worth, and they look to grants and public payers to meet most of their needs.

There are centers which do offer a wide range of services and have a variety of payers. Nonetheless, they still may never be able to generate the revenue necessary to be self-supporting in the general business sense. For them, so many of the patients they see are either uninsured or so poorly insured (with public or private funds) that inadequate revenue can be realized for their services. Outside grants, charity or health system reform which extends coverage to the uninsured may be the only way to ensure the viability of such centers over the long term.

Certainly, if CNCs are to survive, they must seek out, learn about, and help design federal, state, and local public and private funding and insurance mechanisms which pay for nursing services provided at all levels.

Use of Advance Nurse Practitioners

Advanced Nurse Practitioners are employed extensively within CNCs. However, and as already mentioned, they face limitations on where and what type of services they may provide and on whether they will be paid for those services under many insurance and HMO plans.

Certified Nurse Midwives and Certified Registered Nurse Anesthetists reported facing still further constraints through limitations on their clinical privileges in hospitals and other facilities. Even where no laws prohibit their practice, the nurse midwives and nurse anesthetists recounted stories of pressure from the physician community to deny hospital privileges to them or attempts to require the nurses to work for a physician-run practice.

Resistance to and denial of nurse participation on health maintenance organization (HMO) provider panels was even more widely reported. Nurses, no matter what their level of preparation, found roadblocks to practice in a setting that was not supervised or managed by a physician.

Other Advanced Nurse Practitioners did not mention the issue of clinical privileges during the interviews. It is likely, however, that as other ANPs begin to follow their patients across the health continuum and into institutions, they too will face problems with obtaining clinical privileges. Unless the nurse is aligned with the institution(s), opposition will continue or increase as ANPs and CNCs become more visible and competitive.

Centers located in rural areas also complained of the difficulty in simply recruiting and retaining nurses in advanced practice. CNCs face the same opportunities and limitations any rural community faces in trying to attract a provider to its area. Certainly the ANP pay scale ($40,000 plus) demanded by the advanced practice nurse was cited as one drawback for these communities where wages are often lower than in the city.

Pay, however, was also mentioned by those centers trying to recruit from within very large urban areas. Several university centers cited difficulty attracting practitioners because of their salary demands of up to $80,000. Faculty wage structure limited the university's ability to successfully compete or retain ANPs at such a salary.

Competition with Physicians

Providers in communities where CNCs exist do not generally perceive the nursing centers as a competitor or, as in some cases, even know they exist. CNCs frequently focus their efforts on non-paying or low-paying clients, such as Medicaid recipients, and, therefore, are not usually in competition with physicians or others for clients.

Provider perception of a CNC begins to change when a center attempts to include the well-paying or even marginally well-paying insured clients within the practice. Once a CNC seeks out paying clients, the center moves into a competitor role with other local providers. It is also at this point that the CNC must begin to more clearly and effectively market services to clients and other group purchasers of care. If universal health care coverage does become a reality, competition for those previously uninsured but now paying clients will also increase.

Some centers have been able to demonstrate to the local physician community that the CNC actually helps their practices because the center refers clients to them for follow-up. A CNC must be able to document its impact on other providers. The ability to do so, however, is influenced by how large a population the center serves and, therefore, how many people it can refer. Several centers noted they refer nearly 20 percent of their patients to physicians. In addition, winning physician support usually takes at least two to three years.

Licensing and Accreditation

Licensing of CNCs varies by state and program. Corporate structure and the range of services offered dictate what state licenses might be required.

In states such as New York, it is difficult for centers to receive an independent license to operate because of the perceived stringency of requirements for medical direction, equipment, laboratory, and services. In other states, such as Arizona, licensing as an outpatient treatment facility is relatively easy. Still other centers are private practice arrangements and are treated like a physician's practice, with no licensing required except that for a laboratory. Still others are licensed as part of the hospital or other facility with which it might be affiliated (Whitney, Hazen, Fleming, & Swan, 1990).

Like any facility trying to comply with state licensure laws, centers frequently find it difficult and sometimes impossible to obtain independent licenses. Even when they do obtain an independent license, those involved complained of finding the process daunting.

Current literature on the topic does not help very much in clarifying pressing issues. Licensing, certification, and regulation of nursing centers are rarely discussed. These lacks in the literature may be due to the relatively few CNCs in existence and the apparent lack of information about and visibility of them.

Accreditation of CNCs is also very limited. Those centers affiliated with hospitals may enjoy an accreditation status as part of the hospital or part of its ambulatory care program. In this study sample, only birthing centers had sought independent accreditation in an effort to establish credibility and marketability with the public. In addition, birthing centers offer a definable, consistent service to be evaluated. CNCs are not any one type of practice or service and, therefore, present a problem for accreditation and regulation. Reform here is a necessity.

There are accrediting bodies, however, which have programs applicable to community nursing centers. All offer one or another level of accreditation that might apply to a center. Yet, centers usually do not apply because they do not have a medical director, a requirement in many accreditation programs, and one inconsistent with the philosophy and makeup of a nursing center.

A second reason cited for not obtaining accreditation was cost. Unstable centers are reluctant to spend several thousands of dollars for a process that, at present, seems to matter little to the purchaser. The relative invisibility of nursing centers may also account for the lack of any call for a stronger monitoring process. Birthing centers, however, have been extremely visible and in direct competition with hospitals and physicians. To them, accreditation became an issue they had to address. Success here does provide some optimism for the future.

Management and Administration of CNCs

Interviewees perceived centers as nurse started and nurse run, often by nurse faculty, with little or no experience in managing a clinic or practice. The centers were frequently created because of an identified need in the community and the availability of outside funding through federal or private granting bodies. In the eagerness to serve the community and the students, however, little thought was given to how a center becomes or remains financially solvent.

Interestingly, nurses with management experience seem to have been singularly absent in these earlier phases of center development. Although many schools have nursing administration programs, there seems to have been, and continues to be, little effort to link the clinical/practitioner/public health-focused nursing centers with the more hospital-focused nursing administration programs.

Those in private practice stated they did not start with any greater management skills than other centers. What they very quickly realized, however, was that unless they learned how to manage all aspects of their practice, or bought outside assistance, they would not survive. Stories of trial and error both in their own efforts and with those of the consultants they hired predominate. A great hurdle concerned learning to negotiate contracts and payment policies with various consultants, payers, and insurance carriers. Although overall business plans were a rarity, the clear expression of center goals was not; in fact, it was strikingly common. For many, their clear expression of goals guide their practices today as well as they did ten years ago. To improve their level of sophistication in a changing health care market, a number of centers also have recently written business and marketing plans. Let us wish them all success!

Nurses in CNCs find themselves facing many of the same difficulties as physicians. It is difficult for any few providers to mount the administrative, billing, and clinical services necessary to compete effectively in the existing complicated and paper-heavy health care system. Expecting nursing centers to fare any better than physicians who are setting up small practices may not be realistic. The system is making it more and more difficult for any small group of providers to successfully sustain a practice unless they align themselves with a large organizational entity which has or can foster access to numbers of patients.

In general, little effort seems to go into the marketing of services. Some centers suggested that because so many of them serve a poor or disadvantaged population where no other provider is clamoring for clients, they become a provider of choice and therefore marketing is not necessary.

Financing

Birthing centers and CNCs affiliated with a hospital seem to have found it less difficult to tap into capital and operating funds while they struggled in the first year or two of operation. The "parent" offered the "deep pockets" needed until contracts were completed and payments began to flow from private and public payers. For those in their own small business, they operated like most small businesses, taking no income or little income for extended periods of time and capitalizing the businesses from their own pockets.

None of the centers we spoke to were able to obtain bank financing. When they did get loans, it was from individuals who were willing to back them.

Academic centers, on the other hand, seem to experience some level of financial or in-kind support from their institution. Increasingly, however, they are being asked to be self-supporting. Where they are not self-supporting, they are being asked to demonstrate how the center directly benefits the university or the population it serves, beyond that of simply providing an educational experience for students. Still others are being asked by the university to act as a revenue center for the institution.

Space on university campuses does seem to be one benefit often open to centers even with changing demands. Repeatedly, people from academic centers noted that were space allowances to be withdrawn, the center would have to close since revenue was inadequate to cover rent and maintenance. Some community centers face the same situation where local governments and organizations currently provide free space.

Liability Insurance

Birthing centers recounted the greatest difficulty obtaining liability insurance coverage for their centers. Many must insure each practitioner individually rather then through a center policy. Free-standing community centers and those in private practice shared a concern about the ability to obtain liability insurance. The availability of liability insurance at times did limit what, how, where, or if centers provided services.

For many of the academic centers, liability issues were submerged within the larger organization. One center said the attorney for the university was more concerned that someone would get their purse stolen than that the university might be sued for a care-related incident. Most academic centers appear to be covered within the scope of the university's larger policy or self-insurance. The same is true for hospital-affiliated centers and community centers affiliated with a public program.

ACADEMIC CNCs

Mission

In a survey of 65 academic nursing centers in 1988, Zana Higgs reported that most centers had no clear definition or mission except instruction of students. During academic holidays and summer vacations when students or faculty were absent, breaks in service occurred as well. Higgs (1988) concluded that a more consistent balance must be found to meet the needs of students while also providing for the needs of clients.

In response, most fully operational centers now employ full-time or adequate part-time staff to cover operating hours and to avoid breaks in service. However, if staff are funded from grants and grant funding ends, the centers must fall back to faculty and student staffing and decrease operating hours or even close.

Inconsistent or limited operating hours also means a center does not become an integral part of the community's range of health services. It becomes a nice add-on but it does not become a consistent primary provider for the population it is intended to serve. Interviewees stressed that for a center to truly achieve its objectives, it must be integrated into and become part of a stable complement of services offered to the community (Podium, 1993). A faculty or student practice that only operates during the times the school operates cannot accomplish this objective.

Faculty Practice

Overwhelmingly, faculty and deans reported there is no incentive in their system for faculty to engage in practice. If faculty do, it is usually in addition to the rest of their work with no additional pay, even if they generate revenue for the center. Finally, practice is not considered in the efforts to achieve tenure. Time spent in practice actually takes away from time for research and publishing.

Nor was independent faculty practice viewed as useful in terms of securing tenure or promotion. Partially as a result of this approach, several interviewees pointed to a decline in interest in developing centers. In addition, faculty who were involved with the early centers have now moved to other career interests or interests with greater financial and other rewards.

Still, several schools did report on a clinical tract within their programs, similar to those in use in medical schools. One program requires all faculty participating in a center to practice at least one fifth of the time.

Research

Riesch's (1990) empirical literature review includes the history and resurgence of nursing centers and a summary of current research on nursing centers. She concludes that, on the whole, few research studies have been conducted in or about nursing centers, and the existing studies are lacking in many respects. Funding of multisite, multimethod, and clinical trials is proposed to investigate outcomes, cost effectiveness, and quality of care (Riesch, 1990).

Although research is generally thought of in connection with academic settings, the amount of research underway in CNCs does seem limited. Centers have served primarily as sites for nurse practitioner experiences and community service. We were told that, to a limited extent, they have served as research sites. When research has been done, it has usually been of a descriptive nature with little outcome and almost no comparative analysis between centers. Some research has been done on the educational experience, but not on the centers themselves or their products and outcomes or costs. There has been little or no analysis of management practices or comparisons with physician-managed practices.

All those contacted spoke to the need for increased research. This awareness is prompting a more focused research agenda in academic CNCs. Studies have shown advanced practice nurses can provide cost-effective, high-quality primary care (OTA, 1986; Brown & Grimes, 1993; Safriet, 1992; Crosby, Ventura, & Feldman, 1987). Few such studies have been done on the broader nursing care offered from CNCs, but the necessary research is beginning to occur.

CNCs AND CHANGING HEALTH CARE POLICY

Community nursing centers, like many providers operating in a changing health care system, are struggling to find their place. Although many centers reported limitations and difficulties in sustaining their revenue streams, they also reported successes and a growing understanding of how to operate in the system.

Directors identified gaps in their knowledge and skills and are seeking information and assistance to meet them.

As debate continues on health care reform, nurses and nursing centers see themselves as placed firmly within initiatives on prevention and primary care, community-based services, and patient-centered approaches which require educating the consumer to be a more prudent purchaser and user of health care. Unless current health policies are examined for their limitations on non-physician providers, however, nurses and other non-physician care givers will be limited in how well they can respond to the challenge to expand access to care in a revised, or unchanged, health care system. As one interviewee said, "The laws that limit centers are the practice laws that limit nurses."

If nurses (and other non-physician providers) are to help expand access to care for society, they must have access to the settings in which they can see patients for medical or nursing care. Policy makers looking at alternatives to the structure and use of our existing health care system, and the providers within it, must look at whether physician control of practice settings and the flow of payments for care in those settings is still justified in the face of the rapid changes underway in what, how, and where we deliver health care. This approach is called into question particularly when nurses own, manage, or operate a practice/center which needs to receive payment separate from a physician, hospital, or another organization.

Discussions on health care reform by nurses and others refer to the increased role non-physician providers will need to play if the system more aggressively moves toward providing preventive and primary care services. Unless there is significant and rapid expansion of community-based sites which can be used to prepare students and retrain nurses dislocated in a changing system, nursing will be unable to respond to the demand. Facultys of nursing must look beyond the hospital and acute care setting for experiences for all nursing programs.

A SUMMARY OF OBSERVATIONS ON CNCs

Ten observations about the issues facing CNCs are briefly summarized below. Each will require a myriad of professional, public policy, and individual program changes if CNCs are to achieve what we, as nurses, believe we can do to improve health care for the American public.

1. CNCs need to provide a wide range of primary care services offered by nurses and nurse practitioners in order to obtain the revenue necessary to sustain a center.

2. Community-based nursing centers are unable to fulfill their potential as providers of primary care because of limiting federal and state policies, insurance practices, and resistance from physicians.

3. The removal of a number of the limitations confronting centers lies largely in the political arena. Nurses and others interested in expanding the range of reimbursable non-physician provider services will need to challenge the policy makers.

4. Nurses in private practice serve as a bellwether for CNCs by virtue of being the first to confront many of the issues and limitations which will face CNCs as they seek to serve broader segments of the population.

5. CNCs and local physicians can operate cooperatively and use each other as referral sources.

6. When CNCs seek to attract primary care clients covered by private insurance, they enter into direct competition with local physicians. Marketing of CNC services becomes a necessity.

7. Community nursing centers need and want assistance with management skills to allow them to compete more fully and effectively in the health care market place.

8. Preparation of nurses to offer first contact primary care in CNCs is constrained by the limited number of centers, their limited size, and uncertain funding sources.

9. Faculty in schools of nursing have few personal or financial incentives for practice in a CNC yet their participation is crucial if students are to be prepared as primary care providers.

10. There is inadequate research and resources devoted to comparing CNCs and their types of care, management of care, outcomes and costs across centers or against physician management of patients.

REFERENCES

Aydelotte, M. K., Barger, S. E., Branstetter, E., Fehring, R. J., Lindgren, K., Lundeen, S., & Riesch, S. K. (1987). *The nursing center: Concept and design.* Kansas City, MO: American Nurses Association.

Aydelotte, M. K., Hardy, M. A., & Hope, K. P. (1988). *Nurses in private practice.* Kansas City, MO: American Nurses Association.

Brown, S. A., & Grimes, D. E. (1993). A meta-analysis of process of care, clinical outcomes, and cost-effectiveness of nurses in primary care roles: Nurse practitioners and certified nurse-midwives. The American Nurses's Association, Division of Health Policy.

Crosby, F., Ventura, M. R., & Feldman, M. J. (1987). Future research recommendations for establishing NP effectiveness. *Nurse Practitioner, 12,* 75–79.

Higgs, Z. R. (1988). The academic nurse-managed center movement: A survey report. *Journal of Professional Nursing, 4*(6), 422–429.

Office of Technology Assessment (OTA). (1986). Health technology Case Study 37—Nurse practitioners, physician assistant, and certified nurse-midwives: A policy analysis. Congress of the United States, Washington, DC.

Podium. (1993). Nursing centers: A resource to be tapped. An interview with S. Barger. *Syllabus,* American Association of Colleges of Nursing, *19*(3).

Riesch, S. K. (1990). A review of state of the art of research on nursing centers. *Differentiating nursing practice: Into the twenty-first century.* In *Perspectives in nursing: 1989–1991.* New York: National League for Nursing Press.

Riesch, S. K. (1992). Nursing centers: An analysis of the anecdotal literature. *Journal of Professional Nursing, 8*(1), 16–25.

Safriet, B. J. (1992). Health care dollars and regulatory sense: The role of advanced practice nursing. *Yale Journal of Regulation, 9*(2), 417–488.

Sharp, N. (1992). Community nursing centers: Coming of age. *Nursing Management, 23*(8), 18–20.

Whitney, F. W., Hazen, M., Fleming, K., & Swan, B. A. (1990). Three differentiated practice models for ambulatory care. *Differentiating nursing practice: Into the twenty-first century.* In *Perspectives in nursing: 1989–1991.* New York: National League for Nursing Press.

2

*Health Reform
and the Role of
Nursing Centers*

Norman D. Brown

There is nothing more difficult to take in hand, more
perilous to conduct, or more uncertain in its success
than to take the lead in the introduction of a new order of
things.

Machiavelli

FEDERAL AND STATE HEALTH REFORM INITIATIVES

Health reform is not a new issue to American domestic policy makers. Our awareness that something may be fundamentally wrong with the American way of providing medical care has grown steadily more acute. From the Flexner Report to the current chaos of multiple federal bills, health policy in America is a neglected science. It is important to keep in mind that the information discussed in this chapter has been compiled in an ever changing health care reform environment.

Today there are many different legislative initiatives being proposed. As public policy makers struggle to reconcile health care reform issues with the politics of health care, there have been no more comprehensive legislative proposals made public than the proposed Clinton Health Security Act (HSA). In terms of accomplishing universal access to equitably financed, accessible and high-quality health care for all Americans, the HSA should be viewed as a benchmark for deliberations that will lead to a template for formulating comprehensive health reform and not necessarily a final-form piece of legislation.

The Social Security Act of 1935 initially had health reform as one of its principle components. Deleted from the 1935 domestic policy agenda, health reform fulminated for several decades as medical care evolved into the health insurance and fee for service industry. Thirty years after the adoption of the Social Security Act of 1935, the Social Security Act of 1965 established Medicare and Medicaid. There has been relatively little concerted grass roots movement for health care reform—that is until quite recently.

Although the *Health Security Act,* as drafted in the Fall of 1993, has met with extraordinary congressional resistance, it is still a benchmark against which contenders for health reform legislation crown can be measured.

The strengths of the Health Security Act (HSA) include, but are not limited to:

- Guaranteeing universal coverage;
- Working toward equity in the cost of care;
- Fostering the development of comprehensive systems of care in a fragmented health care market place;
- Addressing the issues surrounding planning for the preparation of a diverse health professionals workforce;
- Addressing the issues of role clarification for, and the funding of Outcomes Research utilizing Academic Health Centers;
- Addressing the issues of core public health services, defining, and making a funding priority, essential community providers, including school-based clinics.

The stated purpose of the proposed Clinton Health Security Act was:

> To ensure individual and family security through health care coverage for all Americans in a manner that contains the rate of growth in health care costs and promotes responsible health insurance practices, to promote choice in health care and to ensure and protect the health of all Americans. (Preamble to the Health Security Act 103D Congress, 1st. Session)

The *Health Security Act* (HSA) was comprised of eleven major sections, or Titles. While each of these major sections has some influence on the ways and means that our reformed health care would be configured, specific policies related to the health professions workforce, the role of academic health centers and research priorities for health reform were found in Title III:

> Subtitle A: Workforce Priorities. (HSA, pp. 496–530)
> Subtitle B: Academic Health Centers
> Subtitle C: Health Research Initiative

Subtitle A: Workforce Priorities under Federal Payments

Essentially, this section of the HSA called for, by the academic year 2002–03, no less than 55 percent of physicians in training to be preparing for roles in primary care. This goal would be difficult to attain and should provide more opportunities for nurse/physician collaboration in primary care settings, such as nursing centers. There is another perspective on the number and type of primary care providers which is rapidly emerging.

As we struggle to balance the health care budget, more public policy analysts are realizing the cost effectiveness of utilizing advanced practice nurses (APN). This is particularly true in primary care settings. This trend toward advanced practice nurses providing primary care will have a significant positive impact on the cost of both the education of primary care providers and the appropriate staffing of primary care settings.

Of additional interest to proponents of nursing centers, Section 3061 of Subtitle A addressed the allocation of $200 million for multiple purposes related to the need for, and training of, other licensed providers of health care. While no specific target numbers are cited in terms of trainees, these funds would be partially designated to address the education of nurse practitioners, nurse midwives, BSN level nursing education, curriculum development in community health, and school-based health services, and research related to nursing workforce issues. The need for a program to develop model statutes that remove inappropriate barriers to practice for both nurse practitioners and physician assistants was also noted.

Title III: Section 3061 funds would also support training activities related to Health Administration, research in the effectiveness of managed care, CQI in health care, and research in providing culturally sensitive health care delivery. Funding for continued research in the efficacy of nursing centers could conceivably be derived from this section of the HSA. These funds would also be used for faculty development, trainee support (noted above), other health workforce issues/analysis, the retraining of administrators for jobs as technicians and midlevel providers, and for establishing career planning services, and health professions job banks.

A major feature of HSA-Subtitle A was the establishment of the National Institute for Health Care Workforce Development (HSA: section 3064, p. 528). The Director of this Institute would make recommendations regarding:

- The supply of health care workers needed for the system of regional and Corporate alliance health plans established under Title I of the HSA; and

- The impact of such systems on health care workers and the needs of such workers with respect to the system, including needs regarding education, training, and other matters related to career development. The advisory board of this institute would have as members the Secretary of Labor, the Secretary of Health and Human Services, representatives of health care workers in organized labor, representatives of health care institutions, representatives of health care education organizations, representatives of consumer organizations and others as determined to be appropriate by the Secretaries. This Institute would be phased out at the end of the year 2000.

Subtitle B: Academic Health Centers

This section of the HSA recognized the unique needs of academic medical environments and provided funds for these institutions to continue to meet a variety of purposes. The awarding of these funds to academic health centers may take the form of grants, contracts, and/or cooperative agreements. Academic Health Centers could access these funds to assist with the costs that are not routinely incurred by other entities in providing health services, but are incurred by such centers by the nature of their academic missions.

Other potential sources of revenue for academic health centers were also identified. For example, Academic Health Centers could contract with regional and Corporate alliances to provide specialized treatments (center of excellence concept). Contracts might also be entered into with academic health centers that provide rural information and referral systems.

The funds proposed in section 3103 for health service delivery oriented grants, contracts, and cooperative agreements might not exceed the following amounts (in billions of dollars): 1996—$3.1; 1997 and 1998—$3.2; 1999—$3.7; and 2000—$3.8. In subsequent years, these funds will be adjusted using the "general health care inflation factor." These funds will also be derived from contributions by the Medicare Trust Fund, and the Regional and Corporate Alliances. (The conditions defining payments by the alliances would have been detailed under section 3461 of the Internal Revenue Code of 1986 as added by section 7121 of the HSA (HSA: Subtitle B B, sec 3104).)

Subtitle C: Health Research Initiative

Health Research Initiatives provided academic health centers with directives for research that helped define the research/ scholarship role of academic health centers in the reformed health care environment. Priorities for these scholarly initiatives included the following:

- Research on the effectiveness of alternative clinical strategies, such as, managed care; the quality and outcomes of care, and administrative simplification.
- Research on consumer choice and information resources, the effects of health reform on delivery systems, workplace injury and illness prevention, factors influencing access to health care for underserved populations, and primary care.
- The development of clinical practice guidelines and the effectiveness of such guidelines.

Funding for research initiatives targeting health promotion and disease prevention, which would be available to academic health centers, was proposed at the following levels (in millions of dollars): 1995—$400; 1996 through 2000—$500 each year. Health Services Research would be funded at $150 million in 1995, $400 million in 1996, $500 million in 1997, and in each year from 1998 through 2000 $600 million. Again, for those nursing centers with academic affiliation, these proposed primary care initiatives held promise for promoting research supporting the continued evolution of nursing centers as cost effective and high quality sources of primary care.

STATE LEVEL INITIATIVES

Despite assertions that the states should not wait for federal action, the delay in resolution of the health care reform legislative debate seriously hampered state adoption of reform-minded initiatives. Dr. Marla Salmon recently commented that health reform is a local issue and noted that creativity at the local level is needed to evolve localized cultures of health care into reformed health care environments. While the federal government struggles to delineate its many perspectives on health care reform, today virtually every state has some executive and legislative branch activity focused on the issue of health reform in their unique state health care environment.

The following states have passed some form of Health Reform legislation dealing with insurance reform, alliance formation, and the establishment of some form of state health authority to oversee the implementation of health reform: Florida, Texas, Vermont, Minnesota, Iowa, New Mexico, Ohio, Washington, Virginia, Colorado, and Oklahoma. Most, if not all, states will have active legislation addressing the configuration of the publicly (Medicaid and Medicare) and privately funded health care industry within the 1994/95 biennium.

What health care reform initiatives can we anticipate at the state level? In the near future, legislative sessions will likely include the following subjects:

1. Insurance reform: limits on canceling policies, risk pooling, purchasing cooperatives, and so on.
2. Expansion of practice acts—Nurse Practice Acts to enable nurses to provide services in the full range of their educational preparation.
3. The development of state-wide medical information systems: Cancer registries, Fully Automated Medical Information systems, Hospital discharge data tracking, and other electronic innovations which will facilitate the assessment of individual and aggregated patient outcomes in many dimensions including consumer satisfaction, cost, and effectiveness.
4. Medicaid reform: Movement toward managed care systems and a variety of fiscal practices (capitated, blended, and fee-for-service).
5. The elimination of state legal barriers that are perceived as preventing health care providers from cooperating in joint ventures (i.e., Arkansas city and county-owned hospitals are currently prohibited from joint venturing and developing collaborative networks).

There have been some pretty awkward stutter step attempts at health reform in medicaid managed care at the state level. For example, Tenn Care, Tennessee's managed care medicaid program, has experienced a 2000 doctor resignation from the Tennessee Provider Network. While many of these physicians have since rejoined the network, the primary reason cited for their initial resignation was poor payment schedules. However, lack of autonomy in selecting a caseload and rigid utilization review procedures also add to the frustration of providers. Pete Stark has commented that, "Relying on states to oversee the development of all health reform plans—in the absence of strong federal standards and oversight—will be an unmitigated disaster for consumers."

Nurses should not be embarrassed if they are not knowledgeable about specific health reform initiatives being crafted in each state. It is most appropriate to contact the governor's office and ask to speak with his/her staff person(s) responsible for health care reform initiatives regarding the status of state initiatives. It is important to educate these individuals about ways/means that nurses involved with nursing centers can help meet the demand for accessible, affordable, and high-quality health care that is surely to follow any federal mandate for major reform.

THE ROLE OF NURSING CENTERS IN A REFORMED HEALTH CARE ENVIRONMENT

The fundamental obligations to society of any provider in the reformed health care environment is the provision of services that are consumer centered (i.e., accessible, affordable, and high-quality) and cost effective at the local and national level. "Consumer-centered" refers to providing comprehensive services that are not only the minimum that are federally mandated but those benefits that are to be found in the various health insurance/benefit packages offered in your region. In planning an array of services to be offered through a nursing center, efforts should be made to include services/benefits that are also offered as benefits of a variety of basic service plans. For example, well child check-ups, immunizations, and health-risk appraisals will probably be included in any federally mandated or locally implemented "health plans."

Many of the health services that are needed are also traditionally provided by public health nurses as "gap-filling" services. The following services are among those described as covered medical expenses in the Fall 1993 draft of the HSA and should be of particular interest to nursing center advocates (this is a partial listing of the total covered services):

- Clinical preventive services: An array of primary care/prevention services that include minimum clinical preventive services across the life of the citizen including immunizations, periodic pap/pelvics, mammograms, cholesterol monitoring. At the very least, this benefit assures periodic consumer contact with the health care delivery system.

- Family planning services
- Pregnancy related services
- Hospice
- Home health
- Extended care services
- Ambulance services
- Outpatient rehabilitation
- Durable medical equipment
- Routine vision and hearing exams
- Health education (across the life span)
- Mental health and substance abuse.

Each of these selected benefits can be provided through the efficient utilization nursing centers by nurses who are educationally prepared at a variety of levels. However, knowing the types of services that will be reimbursable alone is not enough to position a nursing center in the main health care revenue streams of their state/region.

COLLABORATIVE PRACTICE/INTEGRATED SYSTEMS OF CARE

The development of collaborative practices with a multitude of other providers is essential for the survival and continued evolution of the nursing center movement. Nursing centers are perfectly positioned to maximize their long practice experience in the provision of primary care and preventive services to not only the disenfranchised, but the mainstream American health care consumer. Among the most fortunate developmental attributes of the traditionally fiscally strapped nursing center movement is the propensity to be efficiently staffed and focused, both in scope of service and cultural appropriateness, in the care they give their communities. Successful nursing centers have collaborative referral arrangements with many different disciplines. This trend toward multidisciplinary team work will continue as the unique value of each profession becomes better defined. The continued evolution of nursing centers will also include opportunities for the development of contractual arrangements for services within the context of larger provider networks.

There have been a plethora of health care system designs that are characterized by their ability to consolidate primary, secondary, and tertiary care into "seamless" networks. These networks are contractual arrangements between a variety of professionals and are tailored to provide consumers with comprehensive care. Usually, participation in a network requires the pooling of capital and may bring some other changes in one's scope of practice. These changes might include reduced practice autonomy, restriction in caseload selection, increased scrutiny of practice guidelines, and increased financial risks. The loss of autonomy can be attributed to the constraints of participating in a joint venture with other professionals. For example, managed care networks often have highly structured caseloads and require detailed utilization review of outcomes for network evaluation. However, for many providers, there are fiscal economies of scale and relative assurance of an active caseload by participating in a network to offset the downside issues.

Nursing centers can be marketed as "building blocks" and components of larger integrated systems of care. In terms of accessibility, nursing centers are traditionally located in a variety of settings, such as churches, schools, community centers, academic settings, and mobile units. They can easily fit the HSA proposed federal definition of a "Preferred Provider," particularly in the following areas:

Primary care/prevention

Family planning

Prenatal care

Well child care/Immunizations

Mental health

Health education.

For example, the appropriateness of a nursing center, as a cradle-to-grave health care resource is particularly clear for providing comprehensive primary care/prevention services. The argument for nursing centers to be included in the design of integrated systems of care is relatively simple—the logic flows in the following way:

If

Primary care/preventive services are desirable covered benefits, and

if nursing center primary care/preventive services are excellent/cost effective and satisfying to consumers,

then

nursing centers should be key components of integrated systems of care and should receive direct reimbursement for these services provided.

The rural and urban settings where nursing centers will thrive in a reformed health care environment include, but are certainly not limited to, senior citizen centers and congregate living centers, homeless shelters, shelters for abused and neglected persons, schools, workplaces, day care centers. Nurses wishing to foster the continued growth of the nursing centers in these and other settings will need to become familiar with the state and local policy makers, gain their confidence, and prove to them the merit of nursing centers in the delivery system.

Nursing center administrators also need to meet with insurance company benefit designers, human service agency directors, and other players in the health care marketplace to educate them about the efficacy of nursing center services.

There is no one right way to venture into a nursing center enterprise with the exception of adhering to a business-like planning process. Academic nursing centers have traditionally had three missions to accomplish: education of students; opportunities for scholarship/faculty practice, and community service. As colleges/schools of nursing realize continued tightening of purse strings, we now must responsibly add revenue generation to the formula for success of any nursing center.

SUMMARY

There has been no better time in this century for nursing to emerge as a key element in providing cost-effective, high-quality, and accessible health care. Nursing centers are "natural" service settings for the provision of primary prevention and primary care services for clients of all ages. Professional nursing must respond to the national health crisis with creative alternatives to the traditional "medical care environment." Collectively, proponents of the nursing center must: stay current with federal and local health reform initiatives; be creative in assessing the potential for providing essential services in your local health care market; collaborate with others in the establishment of integrated systems of care; continue to be attentive to research agendas that support the testing of community based and nursing primary care; and persevere through and actively participate in the turmoil of the next few years as health legislation is drafted and adopted at the federal and state levels.

Nursing has a long history of innovative health services to our country—now is the time that our best creative service delivery ideas can flourish—if we are up to the challenge.

REFERENCES

Brecher, C. (Ed.). (June, 1992). *Implementation issues and national health care reform.* Washington, DC: Josiah Macy Jr. Foundation.

State Health Care Reform Legislation: Public Health Foundation, Washington, DC, 1993.

Health Affairs, Summer, 1992 and Fall, 1993.

3

Evidence in Support of Basing a Nursing Center on Nursing Theory

Ruth M. Neil

If work is all about doing, then the soul is about being:
the indiscriminate enjoyer of everything that comes our
way. If work is the world, then the soul is our home.

D. Whyte, 1994

WHAT'S MISSING IN TOO MANY NURSING CENTERS?

In 1988, Higgs (p. 428) defined nurse-managed-centers as health care systems, organized and managed by nurses. In her survey of academic nurse-managed-centers, she found the services the centers provided and clientele served were based on community needs, curricular needs, and faculty interests. Clinical instruction was identified as the primary purpose for the existence of the centers. Nowhere in her discussion was reference made to using nursing theory as the basis for center operations.

Five years later, Barrett (1993) authored an article entitled "Nursing Centers without Nursing Frameworks: What's Wrong with This Picture?" She argued that nursing centers have the potential for becoming nursing's quintessential contribution to twenty-first century health care, but only if nursing science firmly becomes the basis on which centers offer their services.

Nursing needs to reclaim primary care nursing and differentiate it from primary care medicine. "Primary care nursing is a nursing-care model; primary care medicine is a sickness-cure model" (p. 116).

In this chapter, then, I will offer evidence of the value and success of basing a nursing center on nursing theory—as demonstrated by the Denver Nursing Project in Human Caring (DNPHC or the Caring Center). Included here are strategies for using Watson's (1985, 1988) philosophy and science of human caring as the basis for practice and a discussion of the relationship between theory-based nursing centers and health care reform.

THE CARING CENTER

The Caring Center opened in July 1988 as an outpatient center for clients with human immunodeficiency (HIV) infection/acquired immunodeficiency syndrome (AIDS). It is located in

Denver, Colorado, in Building 5 of the Denver Department of Veterans Affairs Medical Center (DDVAMC). To date, the Center has hosted nearly 22,000 client visits and has served 750 HIV-infected clients, with the current client census being 325.

Sponsorship of DNPHC is shared by DDVAMC, two other local hospitals (University and Denver General), and the University of Colorado School of Nursing, in addition to a Division of Nursing Special Projects Grant. A collaborative agreement details the commitments of each institution to the project in exchange for the care and services provided by the Center for the institutions' HIV-infected clients. Students from the School of Nursing meet some clinical experience requirements at the Center.

Putting "Caring Theory" into Action

Since its inception, DNPHC has been based on Watson's (1985, 1988, 1990) philosophy and science of human caring. As staff have worked together to understand and apply the intent of this framework, it has become evident that this normative theory describes more about "a way of being" than a set of behaviors for nurses "to do."

Major assumptions of Watson's theory are:

1. Caring can be effectively demonstrated and practiced only interpersonally.
2. Caring consists of factors that result in the satisfaction of certain human needs.
3. Effective caring promotes health and individual or family growth.
4. Caring responses accept a person not only as he or she is now, but for what he or she may become.
5. A caring environment offers the development of potential while allowing the person to choose the best action for himself or herself at a given point in time.

6. Caring is more healthogenic than curing. The practice of caring integrates biophysical knowledge with knowledge of human behavior to generate or promote health and to provide ministrations to those who are ill. A science of caring is therefore complementary to the science of curing.

7. The practice of caring is central to nursing (Marriner-Tomey, 1989).

All members of the DNPHC staff are thoroughly oriented and committed to these basic assumptions of the theory and in 1989 developed a mission statement that articulates shared beliefs and values and provides guidance for all Center decisions. Beliefs about the nature of (1) person, (2) health and healing, (3) nursing/caring, and (4) environment, which are common elements of all nursing theories, are the logical core of a nursing organization's mission statement. These beliefs, congruent with Watson's assumptions, are expressed in the DNPHC mission statement and include the following:

1. Every person is unique, has the right and responsibility to make informed choices concerning health, and possesses inner resources and strengths to meet health challenges.

2. Health and well-being are multidimensional, including physical, emotional, mental, spiritual, and social components.

3. Authentic caring relationships between staff and clients encourage self-acceptance, self-love, and self-empowerment.

4. An environment of understanding, love, and concern fosters healing.

(See Appendix for full mission statement.) It seems that over time, each staff member has internalized the theory and "lives it" authentically in relationships not only with clients, but with other staff, students, volunteers, and with other visitors to the Center. A "caring community" has evolved that provides a safe and healing environment for a population of clients living with a life-threatening diagnosis and who often feel misunderstood and stigmatized by society over-all.

Programs and Services

The primary health care available at the Center is multifaceted. Although all clients see a physician or nurse practitioner in the clinic sites of the sponsoring hospitals, their true "partnership" for their primary care develops at DNPHC. Each client is linked with a particular nurse for assistance in maneuvering the many challenges that living with HIV/AIDS can present. The nurses assume special responsibility for their client partners at times of health transition, need for changes in housing, hospitalization, referrals, basic education, and ongoing support. The partnerships exist over time with the clients seeking the guidance and knowledge of "their nurse" in dealing with health issues (Schroeder & Maeve, 1992).

Medically supportive procedures (blood transfusions, lab work, pentamidine treatments, and others) are carried out at the Center as are numerous complementary healing options (massage, Reiki, reflexology, art and writing therapy, and meditative practices). A wide range of individual and group education and emotional support services are also offered.

THE NURSING CENTER
AS A COMMUNITY

The shared values and beliefs grounded in Watson's theory create a solid foundation for community. The mission statement is periodically reviewed by all staff and is publicly posted and becomes part of the consciousness of clients and other Center participants as well. "DNPHC is a very popular 'drop-in' place. Numerous clients spend time at the Center each day, just to talk with people, to enjoy the feeling of belonging somewhere, sometimes to take a nap or wait for a prescription to be filled" (Neil, 1994). The relevance and need for this kind of environment is no doubt more pronounced for persons living with HIV/AIDS than persons with other health-related problems. The "freedom" inherent in Watson's theory that encourages such an environment is therefore especially well-suited for meeting the needs of this population.

In addition to shared values and beliefs, a community depends on open and honest communication. Center staff learned early that to truly honor and "live out" the theory, they needed to accept responsibility to communicate with each other in this manner. Various strategies have been implemented to increase mutual respect among staff members and to facilitate their ability to support and care for one another. The result has been a highly empowered, self-directed, professionally satisfied staff with no turnover for nearly two years (NLN, 1994).

In addition to the informal "drop-in" visits and free Friday lunches, scheduled visits for medically supportive care, nursing support, counseling, education, referral, and complementary healing options, clients participate in the organizational life of the Center as well. A Client Advisory Committee meets bimonthly and serves as the official liaison between staff and the client population in making decisions regarding services, policies, and programs. Clients conduct fund-raising projects to maintain and administer a Client Emergency Fund. Clients participate in volunteer and paid work opportunities that (a) support the work of the Center, (b) result in the monthly newsletter, and (c) add meaning and a sense of belonging to the lives of the clients. (The paid work program is funded annually by a grant from a local trust.)

HAS IT ALL MADE A DIFFERENCE?

Numerous methods have been used to document and evaluate outcomes of DNPHC's overall program as well as individual caring activities. Central to caring theory is the belief that the definition of a "positive outcome" must incorporate the client's values and goals. The "community" characteristics of DNPHC described foster open communication between clients and staff on a continuing basis, and the Center's relatively small size allows for quick "self-correction" of programs or policies that are not effective.

Monthly records, kept since the Center opened in 1988, indicate steady growth in use of the Center and a continually increasing client census, even though client deaths occur at the rate of approximately 1.5 per week. Formal program evaluation has been accomplished through focus groups (Schroeder & Neil, 1992), and periodic written questionnaires (Schroeder, 1993; Schroeder & Maeve, 1992).

Data analysis completed for the calendar years 1991 and 1992 indicates that client use of DNPHC contributes to cost savings for the sponsoring institutions through prevented or shortened hospitalizations, provision of outpatient medically supportive treatments, more effective use of other resources (through referral) available in the community, and improved sense of empowerment and quality of life from the clients' perspectives. The amount of savings to the three hospitals for 1991 was calculated to be $700,000 and for 1992, $1,100,000 (Schroeder, 1993). Similar analysis is currently being conducted for 1993. Since the three hospitals involved are obligated to provide care to this uninsured or underinsured population, their interest in doing so as cost-effectively as possible promotes their continuing support of the Center.

Unsolicited "outcome evaluation" comes in periodic spontaneous donations from various individuals, agencies, and organizations, the generous service of volunteers (massage, Reiki, and reflexology therapists, professional support group facilitators, office support staff, and assistance with the Friday lunch program), and the receipt of six separate awards for excellence in services to the HIV/AIDS community. The appreciation expressed by clients who use DNPHC (and their families and friends) continues to be the most personal and rewarding documentation of positive outcome. One typical example was a recent letter written by the wife of a client. Her letter includes the following words: "My husband acquired AIDS through a blood transfusion. To have this disease is like living in a nightmare. People are afraid of you. Your friends are not your friends anymore. When we found the Caring Center, it was like we finally got fresh air. The staff couldn't be any better if God himself were down here to do it. I am a mother of six grown children, but they cannot give me the support that I get at the Caring Center."

RELATIONSHIP TO HEALTH CARE REFORM

Caring theory-based nursing as provided at DNPHC is an augmentation model for primary health care delivery, not a substitute medical model. Barrett (1993) pointed out that primary health care is a cornerstone of most existing nursing centers. "Unfortunately, there is a danger that primary health care may become a euphemism for primary care medicine, just as health care has become a euphemism for medical care" (p. 116). This observation underscores the necessity for nursing science/ theory to be deliberately chosen as the framework for nursing centers. In this way, the public will have the opportunity to observe and appreciate *what is uniquely nursing* and, in time, truly want health care reform that features and values nursing's approach to primary health care which, historically, has been community-based and empowering for the individual. As was recently observed by a well-known health policy and ethics expert, "What we see being proposed by Washington is not health care reform. Rather, it is medical reimbursement reform." Unless nurses unite in their commitment to offer a real alternative to the current medical care "system," the public and policy-makers will not have access to nursing's vision for true change.

"Theories may be thought of as mechanisms to facilitate nursing practice, as guiding lights that illuminate the path to nursing empowerment, which operationalize plans to bring about desired outcomes in patients, in practice, and in health care settings" (Sorrentino, 1991, p. 54). As a practice discipline, nursing has a responsibility to provide quality care based on a body of knowledge generated and tested through the process of reflective practice and scientific inquiry. Nursing centers provide the ideal setting for refining and enhancing nursing theory and for showcasing what nursing truly is for a society that needs a new vision about health care.

Barrett (1993) pointed out that grassroots efforts by nurses in practice, education, and research are essential to change nursing's public image. Although lengthy, her suggestions are worthy of inclusion. Nurses' efforts need to include:

1. Voicing revolutionary cries for people-centered systems.

2. Communicating with the public by talking about what nursing is and what it is not while clarifying the important, yet different contributions of various disciplines to clients' overall personal health care agenda.

3. Enhancing consumer power through advocacy, health care education, and increasing awareness of the benefits of nursing care.

4. Organizing and participation in think tanks designed to operationalize proposals such as the Pew Commission's Competencies for Future Health Providers from a nursing science perspective that reflect the way different nursing frameworks interpret our disciplinary uniqueness.

5. Formulating health care policy, services, and practices that are informed by consumer voices not ordinarily heard and informed by nursing science knowledge.

6. Putting clients in the center of decision making by giving them the necessary information to participate knowingly.

7. Advocating legislation requiring nursing frameworks as the scientific basis for nursing centers.

8. And, lastly, preparing to resist backlash. (p. 117)

DISCUSSION

The Denver Nursing Project in Human Caring seems to measure up well against the challenging agenda set forth by Barrett. The consistent quality and excellence that grows out of a conscious and conscientious commitment to Watson's philosophy and science of human caring is supported in client satisfaction with care, enhanced quality of life, an empowered, autonomous, and fulfilled staff, and cost savings to sponsoring agencies.

Even with this record of success, the funding challenges continue. Health (medical) care financing systems continue to invest more heavily in the high-cost intensive technological and pharmacologic services than the lower-cost health-promoting, healing, and self-empowering opportunities provided by nursing.

The experiences of persons living with HIV/AIDS have much to teach the larger society, especially in relation to questions of health care reform. Care providers working with this population (physicians, social workers, psychologists, occupational therapists, nurses, and others) have all been challenged to reexamine the nature of the provider-client relationship and adopt a model of "partnership" in contrast to the traditional paternalistic approach. This factor in itself offers an improved vision of what a reformed health care system could look like.

In addition, the experience of growth and healing that occurs for many HIV/AIDS clients, even as their physical bodies deteriorate and die, provides a more realistic definition of health/illness. Lamendola and Newman (1994) recently wrote of AIDS as expanding consciousness, demonstrating again the vision of nursing's broad and enlightened conceptual framework to encompass and explain complex truths about human nature and provide guidance for health-oriented outcomes. Contemporary society, faced with a myriad of problems ranging from violence and abuse to homelessness and poverty, needs and deserves the vision and guidance available in nursing theories, not only in dealing with health/illness issues, but in creating more caring communities for all aspects of life. What better place to see these theories being modeled, than in nursing centers?

REFERENCES

Barrett, E. A. M. (1993). Nursing centers without nursing frameworks: What's wrong with this picture? *Nursing Science Quarterly,* 6(3), Fall, 115–117.

Higgs, Z. R. (1988). The academic nurse-managed center movement: A survey report. *Journal of Professional Nursing,* 4(6), November–December, 422–429.

Lamendola, F. P., & Newman, M. A. (1994). The paradox of HIV/AIDS as expanding consciousness. *Advances in Nursing Science,* 16(3), 13–21.

Marriner-Tomey, A. (1989). *Nursing theorists and their work.* Toronto: C.V. Mosby Co.

National League for Nursing (1994). *A guide to applying the art and science of human caring* (Videotape series and accompanying monograph). New York: Author.

Neil, R. M. (1994). Authentic caring: The sensible answer for clients and staff dealing with HIV/AIDS. *Nursing Administration Quarterly,* 18(2), 36–40.

Schroeder, C. A. (1993). Nursing's response to the crisis of access, costs, and quality in health care. *Advances in Nursing Science,* 16(1), 1–20.

Schroeder, C. A., & Maeve, M. K. (1992). Nursing care partnerships at the Denver Nursing Project in Human Caring: An application and extension of caring theory in practice. *Advances in Nursing Science,* 15(2), 25–38.

Schroeder, C. A., & Neil, R. M. (1992). Focus groups: a humanistic means of evaluating an HIV/AIDS program based on caring theory. *Journal of Clinical Nursing,* 1, 265–274.

Sorrentino, E. A. (1991). Making theories work for you. *Nursing Administration Quarterly,* 15(1), 54–59.

Watson, M. J. (1985). *Nursing: The philosophy and science of caring.* Boulder, CO: Colorado Associated University Press.

Watson, M. J. (1988). *Nursing: Human science and human care.* New York: National League for Nursing.

Watson, M. J. (1990). Transpersonal caring: A transcendent view of person, health, and healing. In M. W. Parker (Ed.), *Nursing theories in practice* (pp. 277–288). New York: National League for Nursing.

APPENDIX

THE CARING CENTER

The Denver Nursing Project in Human Caring (Caring Center) is an outpatient center dedicated to offering comprehensive nursing services, authentically and responsibly, to persons infected and affected by HIV/AIDS in an environment where the dignity and uniqueness of each individual is honored and respected.

Mission Statement

The first mission and top priority of the The Denver Nursing Project in Human Caring is facilitation of high quality health care to HIV-positive clients and their lovers, friends, families and designated others who make up their support systems. Such health care is based on respect for each person and belief that health and wellbeing are multidimensional—including physical, emotional, mental, spiritual and social components. Every person is unique and has the right and responsibility to make informed choices concerning health. Each also possesses inner resources and strengths to meet health challenges. Through establishment of authentic caring relationships, the DNPHC staff and clients encourage self-acceptance, self-love, and self-empowerment. The staff belief is that the healing process is fostered by the understanding, love, and concern of those who care.

Education is the second mission of the DNPHC. Education is the foundation for competent care of others as well as care of oneself. Clients and staff continue to share openly their knowledge and experience as greater understanding develops about the spectrum of HIV-induced health changes. DNPHC staff and clients also serve as resource persons for various education programs in the community. In addition to client and family education, training and observational programs for students and professionals from nursing and other health-related disciplines are provided at the Center.

The third mission of the DNPHC is to foster professional health care practices based on research findings. This includes staying abreast of the professional literature, participating in research conferences, initiating nursing research, and cooperating with other disciplines and agencies as appropriate in the conduct of research. DNPHC is also committed to demonstrating and disseminating information regarding the cost effectiveness of the nursing center model.

Nursing practices carried out at the DNPHC are based on Jean Watson's theory of Human Care Nursing. This provides opportunity for ongoing validation of the theory as well as basis for research questions.

4

Information Systems for Community Nursing Centers: Issues of Clinical Documentation

Sally Peck Lundeen

If you keep doing what you are already doing, you will keep getting what you've already got.

Ted Gaebler

SALLY PECK LUNDEEN

*T*here are many management information system applications available to community nursing centers (CNCs) in today's technological environment. In addition to ever more sophisticated word processing, desktop publishing, and graphics programs, dozens of computerized systems have been developed to support the office management functions of appointment scheduling and follow-up, client tracking, staffing, and billing. Many other clinically focused programs support clinical decision making, long distance consultation and education, health professionals' education, and client teaching. Finally, there are numerous systems on the market that organize clinical data and even generate the clinical record.

Perhaps the most important and least well developed of the information system applications essential to Community Nursing Centers (CNCs) is the clinical documentation systems. In the face of the rapidly expanding technology in this area and the plethora of systems being developed and marketed to a promising ambulatory care market, it is easy to become confused about which system will best support the clinical documentation needs of community nursing centers. The implementation of a clinical information system is a very costly undertaking in any setting, both in the allocation of fiscal funds and human resources. It is critical that CNC administrators define clearly the purpose(s) for which clinical data will be used in their particular setting so as to purchase or develop systems that are able to support these needs. Both immediate and long-term goals must be considered if the appropriate fit is to be developed between the clinical practice setting and the clinical data system. The best choice will always be an MIS system that can grow with the changing needs of the CNC over time.

The purpose of this chapter is to (a) review the utility of computerized information systems for Community Nursing Centers; (b) identify some key questions that CNC information systems should address; and (c) suggest the potential of adopting common data elements for CNCs as the basis for relational clinical documentation system development.

THE UTILITY OF COMPUTERIZED INFORMATION SYSTEMS FOR CNCs

The systematic collection and reporting of accurate administrative and clinical information in CNCs is critical. Efficient and effective center management demands the ability to review data related to client utilization patterns, staffing patterns, resource allocation, and costs. Reimbursement or support by external funders relies heavily on the ability of CNCs to keep and report accurate client- and service-related data. It is essential to have a mechanism to collect and store clinical data in order to monitor the process and quality of care. Finally, there is a mandate for clear and accurate clinical documentation since the clinical record stands as a legal document.

The need to collect, store, and analyze data is shared by CNCs and nearly all other health care service providers. Most health care settings use computers to simplify the management of large amounts of data. The need to develop computerized information systems that include clinical data for community nursing centers far surpasses the mere convenience and efficiency espoused by enthusiasts, however. In addition to the need to produce information in the basic reporting categories, many CNCs also have an interest in collecting and analyzing data related to research, health professionals education, and health policy. In fact, as change-oriented organizations facing a struggle for survival, CNCs are more likely than stable, long-standing institutions to rely on the documentation of both process and outcome data in order to make a case for long-term viability.

In spite of the fact that CNCs are frequently small organizations, the nature of their data management requirements are no less complex that organizations many times their size. "Off the shelf" products developed for other clinical settings are unlikely to be sophisticated enough to meet the multiple needs of CNCs. Moving beyond reimbursement and office management software applications to include the development of computerized clinical information systems appropriate for CNCs is necessary not only to support the multiple goals of CNCs, but to insure their very survival.

RELATIONAL DATABASES FOR CLINICAL INFORMATION SYSTEMS

To provide the answers to key questions related to the management of CNCs, the assurance of quality services, the education of health professionals, issues of interest to researchers, and outcome data of interest to policy makers, clinical information systems must be constructed as relational databases. That is, the various data elements in the system must be able to be related to each other in order to provide answers to complex questions. For instance, billing data is necessary but not sufficient to answer policy-related questions about the nature of reimbursement policy and practices related to primary prevention and other nursing interventions (i.e., health teaching, guidance and counseling, and case management). Billing data must be linked in the system to various client and clinical data elements.

Although the programming of information systems to structure the relationships necessary to link data elements is generally the role of MIS specialists, the conceptualization of the framework necessary to define the appropriate links must be the role of clear thinking providers. In the case of clinical information systems for CNCs, professional nurses who are involved in the development and implementation of clinical delivery models must also be actively involved in the development of new information systems that will support and adequately reflect these evolving practice models. Successful communication and collaboration between these two disciplines is most likely to result in the new clinical documentation systems needed for community nursing centers.

We cannot rely on information systems that have been developed for other clinical settings or providers, if we continue to assert that there is something unique about CNC settings. Therefore, existing systems must be evaluated and new systems developed using a community nursing center framework. Information systems that have served ambulatory medical care systems well are conceptualized around medical practice models. These systems are not adequate to support the practice models being developed by CNCs who use nursing models of care (ANA, 1987) with an emphasis on health promotion and disease prevention, and consumer-focused supportive services. If CNCs are truly different in some ways from primary care medical clinics, their clinical information systems must reflect the differences as well as the similarities. This suggests that nursing taxonomies must be included to document nursing care.

A modification of the old management information system adage "garbage in—garbage out" also deserves some thought. That is, one must define the questions of interest before system development if you expect answers after system implementation. Although this seems an obvious cautionary note, the conceptual basis for an MIS system is frequently not adequately delineated during the development or evaluation of a system. Proof of this observation lies in the number of very expensive and complex clinical data systems in existence (and currently under development) that are unable to answer very basic questions related to both professional practice and client outcomes.

What are the questions that we need to answer about community nursing centers that our information systems should help us address? In short, we need to be able to describe our clients—who are they and what needs do they present? We need to be able to describe our practice—what do we do and how do we do it? We need to be able to describe outcomes— what difference does it make? We need to be able to determine the allocation of resources—what does it cost? We need to be able to share the answers to the first four questions with others—what and how do we teach what we have learned?

Management questions, clinical questions, research questions, educational questions, and policy questions can be reduced to these four basic categories. The specific questions that need to be addressed by specific CNCs will vary, however, based on the nature of the community being served and the nature of the practice model being developed. The mission, goals and objectives, and the organizational structure of CNCs vary also. This may cause more or less emphasis to be placed on each of these basic questions in each setting. Information management systems must be designed with the flexibility to allow each CNC staff to answer the questions of most relevance to them.

In addition, these categories of questions are clearly not mutually exclusive. The ability to link data relationally between the categories of client descriptors, provider process, and cost is critical to our ability to generate the answers to research, educational and policy questions related to community nursing centers. Computerized information systems for CNCs must include clinical documentation and client descriptor data as well as management and billing data information and these data elements must be relationally linked if the systems are to respond to the evolving information and data analysis needs of these centers.

COMMON DATA ELEMENTS FOR CNC INFORMATION SYSTEMS

The number of community nursing centers seems to be growing (Barger & Rosenfeld, 1993) and the nature of these primary health care models is consistent with a trend in public policy toward more community-based, primary prevention focused delivery strategies. However, to date there has been minimal inclusion of CNCs per se in the health care reform debate or in the literature on integrated delivery systems. In fact, although at the forefront of health care reform in many ways, CNCs for the most part are still operated as small, independent businesses or as the service units of schools and colleges of nursing. Most CNCs struggle financially and few survive solely on revenue from traditional financing streams.

It can be argued that CNCs will never play a significant role in the improvement of access to care and health status until public policies related to the definition of a basic package of "covered" health care services and compensation for providers delivering those services are changed. It can also be argued that CNCs as an evolving delivery model can play a significant role in redefining how primary health care is both delivered and paid for. In order to assume this leadership role, CNCs must be shown to have both a positive impact on the health outcomes of users and a positive influence on overall health care costs. The research necessary to have an impact on policy makers in these areas is not possible without the collection and analysis of large CNC datasets. Nurses who operate community nursing centers must be able to clearly define who our clients are and the specific nature of our interventions. We must commit to the documentation and evaluation of program outcomes. We must be able to document the impact of our interventions with different aggregate groups over time. We must be able to determine our costs and project our potential cost savings to the system. This key research agenda will be immeasurably strengthened through the systematic collection of nursing data.

Nurses advocating the support and expansion of CNC models as a part of health care reform are more likely to have an impact on changes in health policy if we are armed with scientifically sound studies on the impact of nursing practice models on these factors. These studies must be based on multiple site comparisons of CNC models and strategies. Such studies are not possible without the collection of common data elements in many nursing center settings.

Werley and colleagues (Werley & Lang, 1988; Werley, Devine, & Zorn, 1989) have long argued for a Nursing Minimum Data Set (NMDS) that would provide a common dataset across many nursing practice settings. Documentation of clinical practice using a NMDS framework is based on one of several available nursing taxonomies (Carpentino, 1991; McCloskey & Bulechek, 1992; Martin & Scheet, 1992; Saba, 1992). Developmental work is underway to develop and test CNC information systems that use a relational database platform and a nursing taxonomy as the clinical documentation system (Lundeen & Friedbacher, 1994).

Using the NMDS framework, the MIS Workgroup of the NLN Nursing Center Council is currently working toward consensus on a set of core data elements to recommend as a basis for CNC information system development across settings. A critical mass of CNCs must agree to collect these core data elements (commonly defined) if the necessary multiple site health services research studies are to be conducted. Continuing work in this area supports a key goal of the current Council for Nursing Centers and will serve as the basis for continuing policy development toward health care reform.

SUMMARY

The need for community nursing centers to implement clinical information frameworks as a part of MIS development is critical to the success and perhaps the very survival of the these innovative primary care delivery models. The challenge to CNC leaders is to develop clinical documentation systems that are based on nursing models of care and provide for the documentation of nursing interventions. This will require the utilization of nursing taxonomies in the development of these systems in addition to the use of the medical labels currently necessary for reimbursement of services. Nurses in CNCs must participate in building a consensus on the common data elements to include in these information systems and the relational linkages appropriate to answer the research and policy questions of concern. The potential for CNCs to demonstrate effectiveness as unique and important settings in a restructured delivery system may depend on the extent to which we are successful in this endeavor.

REFERENCES

American Nurses Association. (1987). *The nursing center: Concept & design.* (Publication #CH-17). Kansas City, MO: Author.

Barger, S., & Rosenfeld, P. (1993). Models in community health care. *Nursing & Health Care, 14*(8), 426–431.

Carpentino, L. (1991). *Nursing care plans and documentation: Nursing diagnoses and collaborative problems.* Philadelphia: Lippincott Co.

Lundeen, S. P., & Friedbacher, B. E. (1994). The automated community health information system (ACHIS): A relational database application of the Omaha system in a community nursing center. In S. J. Frobe & E. S. P. Puyter-Wenting (Eds.), *Nursing informatics: An international overview for nursing a technological era* (pp. 393–397). Amsterdam: Elsevier.

Martin, K. S., & Scheet, N. J. (1992). *The Omaha system: Applications for community health nursing.* Philadelphia: W. B. Saunders Co.

McCloskey, J. C., & Bulechek, G. M. (Eds.). (1992). *Nursing interventions classification (NIC).* St. Louis: Mosby-Year Book.

Saba, V. K. (1992). The classification of home health care nursing diagnoses and interventions. *Caring, 11*(3), 50–57.

Werley, H. H., Devine, E. C., & Zorn, C. R. (1989). Nursing minimum data set: An abstraction tool for computerized nursing services data. In V. K. Saba, K. A. Rieder, & D. B. Pocklington (Eds.), *Nursing and computers: An anthology* (pp. 191–193). New York: Springer-Verlag.

Werley, H. H., & Lang, N. M. (Eds.). (1988). *Identification of the nursing minimum data set.* New York: Springer.

5

Community Nursing Center Informatics for Business, Practice, Research, and Education

Patricia Hinton Walker
John M. Walker

A person's judgment cannot be better than the information upon which it is based.
Arthur Hayes Sulzberger, 1948

*C*ommunity nursing centers (CNCs) have the potential to play a very significant role in health care reform. However, these relatively new organizations must attend to their information needs in order to survive in an increasingly competitive health care delivery market. As organizations become more competitive, they must begin to control and understand their own data, information, and business processes. This chapter presents a comprehensive method of planning for the development of needed information systems and the purchase and/or design of business software to support the various functions of community nursing centers.

The University of Rochester CNC is an innovative, comprehensive nursing center with a number of satellite faculty practices in urban and rural areas. Service clusters were developed and marketed that include Life Transitions and Developmental Changes; Organizations, Business and Health Care Providers; Longer Term Continuity of Care; and Life Altering Crisis (Walker, 1991, p. 19). This CNC was developed in the spirit of "unification," consequently education, practice, and research interests and needs must be addressed. In addition, this CNC was developed as a professional corporation and functions as a small entrepreneurial business. The development of a comprehensive plan for an information system was needed to support an academic nursing center like the University of Rochester School of Nursing CNC.

Organizations that lack a planned strategy or methods and procedures for obtaining appropriate information technology end up with fragmented, incompatible communications and computer systems. Consequently, an organization frequently experiences poor use of its own data. Without strategically linked planning of information technology, there is often data entry redundancy or incompatibility with other systems and software within the same organization. This complicates critical business processes and can even result in confusion and inefficiencies due to unreliable, inappropriate, or inaccurate data.

The basic principle behind Information Resource Management contends that, "Information is a corporate resource and should be planned on a corporate-wide basis regardless of the fact that it is used in many different computers and departments" (Martin, 1990a, p. 15). This statement was particularly true for the University of Rochester CNC, which was developed as a "center without walls." The information needs requirements were diverse in nature and required the use of computer hardware and software at CNC offices and in many satellite faculty practice sites. Also critical for this nursing center was the development of systems that would facilitate data collection, management, and analysis to support the business, practice, research, and education functions of the CNC. "Many top executives believe that by the mid-1990s, more than 90 percent of all U.S. jobs will be information- or service-related, compared with 60 percent during the 1940s" (Coleman & Cullinane, 1991, p. 309).

Development of a nursing center as a computerized corporation with a systematic plan for information systems for the Rochester CNC required the use of information engineering. This term implies "top-down planning, data modeling, and function process modeling of the enterprise as a whole rather than to isolated projects" (Martin, 1990a, p. 15). Most nursing leaders and managers are familiar with strategic planning and business planning for organizations; however, for information systems, information strategy planning is required for development of a comprehensive plan for integrated information systems.

INFORMATION STRATEGY PLANNING

The information strategy planning process, according to Martin (1990a, pp. 13–15) has six components:

1. Analysis of goals and problems;
2. Critical success factor analysis;
3. Technology impact analysis;

4. Strategic systems vision;

5. An overview model of the functions of the enterprise, and

6. Entity-relationship modeling.

McFadden and Hoffer (1991, p. 141) suggest seven similar steps. Only three components of information systems planning will be highlighted for the purposes of this chapter:

1. Critical success factors,

2. Overview modeling which includes function modeling and,

3. Entity-relationship modeling, which is important to CNCs with research goals.

The information strategy planning process is usually approached in two distinctive layers. The first and top layer is usually obtained from top managers and relates to the vision, goals, and future impact of technology on an organization and factors critical to the success of the organization. The second and more detailed layer of the information strategy planning process involves modeling of the enterprise, its functions, its activities, and its data and information needs.

Critical Success Factors

Critical success factors, according to Martin (1990b, p. 581) are defined as, "An internal or external business-related result that is measurable and that will have a major influence on whether a business segment meets its goals." Critical success factors are sometimes referred to as the key areas where things must go right for the organization to succeed in accomplishing its goals. According to Martin (1990a, p. 14), critical success factor analysis "identifies critical assumptions that need checking, critical information needs, and critical decisions for which decision-support systems are needed."

For the University of Rochester CNC, six critical success factors were identified that would drive the information strategy planning process. Critical success factors identified by the CNC director in consultation with CNC faculty members were:

1. Development of diverse revenue streams;
2. Cost control;
3. Providing and documenting quality services (care);
4. Client and faculty practitioner satisfaction;
5. Development of practice-based research; and
6. Integration of the CNC into the educational activities of the school of nursing.

Based on concern reflected in the nursing literature about the financial viability of nursing centers, especially those relying on grant funding or third-party reimbursement, the first two factors were critical just for survival. Next, nursing centers must demonstrate the ability to provide safe, quality nursing services to the community. If quality care is provided in a customer-sensitive way, the client will be satisfied. It is equally critical however, that the faculty practitioner be satisfied with the faculty practice role. There are numerous examples in the nursing literature of the frustrations of faculty who practice. Consequently, in order to continue to grow, academic nursing centers must develop organizational structures that support practicing faculty members.

Once the CNC practices are financially supported, quality care is being provided, and the customer/provider is satisfied with the services, then nursing center administrators can pay attention to the contributions that nursing centers can make to the professional community. Practice-based research must be developed to demonstrate the effectiveness of nurse-managed care to underserved populations. This research will provide not only additional financial support for new and innovative activities, but the health policy implications are critical to the long-term survival of nursing centers. Because research is a major emphasis within the University of Rochester School of Nursing, this is an internal critical success factor.

Nursing centers offer important new opportunities for students to be educated in community-based settings. Advance practice nurses in nursing centers who are providing care for underserved populations in urban and rural settings serve as important role models for nursing students of the future. With health reform and the shift in health care delivery to the community, integration of CNC practices into the educational mission of the school of nursing is also a critical success factor. CNC practice sites can provide futuristic clinical experiences for students at all levels in the curriculum. Since the University of Rochester CNC was established as a business model, with faculty practice as the primary purpose, the critical success factors were determined in this order. Nursing centers in other types of institutions might choose different critical success factors or set different priorities depending on mission, goals, and the parent institution.

BUSINESS FUNCTION MODELING

The goal of business function modeling is to analyze basic business functions, processes, and activities of the organization, and to identify present/future information needs to support these functions. For in-depth treatments of business function modeling, see McFadden and Hoffer, (1991, p. 47) and Martin (1990a, p. 43). "A business function is a group of activities which together support one aspect of furthering the mission of the enterprise" (Martin, 1990a, p. 43). Business functions as described by McFadden and Hoffer (1991, p. 148) are, ". . . broad groups of closely related activities and decisions that contribute to a product or service life cycle."

The CNC functions were identified after much thought and consideration. This is an important first step that CNC administrators who are planning an information system must carefully think through. Consistent with the mission of the University of Rochester, (education, practice, and research) the major functions of this CNC are:

1. Development of faculty practice roles/opportunities;
2. Education of students; and
3. Conducting research (see Figure 1).

Since the CNC is also organized as a professional corporation that is a business, there are additional functions critical to the survival of the organization. These include administrative functions such as scheduling, project management, administration of the faculty members practicing in the community, telecomputing, providing clerical support, and communication internally in the school and externally in the community. Business functions also included the key components of financial management (planning, budgeting, projecting, and accounting), and the development of entrepreneurs. (See Figures 1 and 2.)

Other information that would assist the novice in determining the business functions of their particular organization are provided by Martin (1990a, p. 43). He indicates that, "A function is ongoing and continuous; a function is not based on organizational structures; a function categorizes what is done, not how" (Martin, 1990a, p. 54). How things get done is related to the procedures.

Processes and procedures are different within business function modeling. *Procedures* are organizationally required activities that are needed to conduct a process. A corporate decision to use a particular software package for a particular process to support a business function could be part of the procedure required to get the job done efficiently.

Organizational functions can be subdivided into processes. For example, for the business function *financial management,* four processes were identified for CNC purposes: planning, budgeting, projecting, and accounting. McFadden and Hoffer (1991, p. 148) state that business processes are "decision-related

Figure 1 Administrative function model.

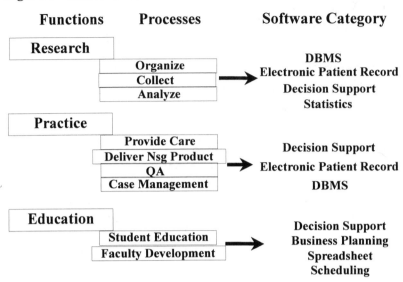

activities that occur within a function and often serve to manage people, money, material, or information. Whereas a function is ongoing and continuous, a process relates to a specific act that has definable beginning and ending points. A process has identifiable inputs and outputs" (Martin, 1990a, p. 43).

The next step in business function modeling is to identify the processes for each of the business functions of the CNC and begin to determine software (or types of software) needed as part of the information system. The business functions and processes of the CNC were identified and divided into two major groups. One function/process grouping was related to *administrative, financial,* and *entrepreneurial* actions that are depicted in Figures 2 and 3. The second group, functions related to the *practice, education,* and *research* mission of the CNC is demonstrated in Figure 1 which relates to the practice, education, and research functions of the parent organization, the University of Rochester School of Nursing.

Figure 2 Business function model.

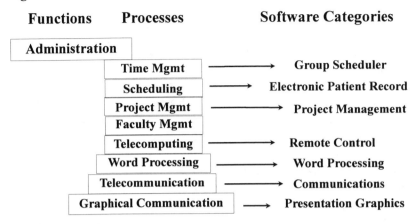

Figure 3 CNC functions.

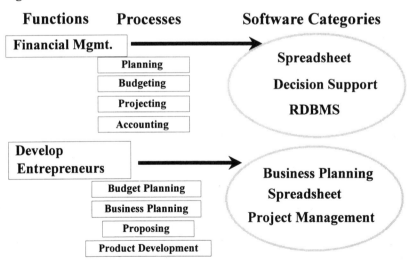

SUPPORT FOR ADMINISTRATIVE AND BUSINESS-RELATED FUNCTIONS

According to Potash and Taylor (1993), there are four types of faculty practice organizations: unification, collaboration, the integrated model, and the entrepreneurial model. Unification is described at the University of Rochester and Rush Presbyterian, where administration of clinical agencies and the school of nursing are "unified" and faculty members practice as clinicians and are also educators. However, with the entrepreneurial model, there is support for faculty members who design their own faculty practices that should also provide opportunities for teaching or research. The University of Rochester CNC, although it is conceptually housed within a unification structure, is an entrepreneurial faculty practice organization.

In addition to being an entrepreneurial organization (as mentioned previously) the CNC was managed as a small business. The first critical success factor is related to development of sound administrative and financial management functions and requires management of costs for survival of the organization. Consequently, the selection of CNC administrative and business-related software was extremely important. Figures 2 and 3 show the processes contained within the administrative, financial management, and development of entrepreneurs functions and identify the respective software categories required to support any CNC that is managed as a business.

These processes under *administration* include activities, such as scheduling, time management, management of the faculty, and their respective satellite faculty practices. In the important area of *financial management*, processes such as financial planning, budgeting, forecasting, or projecting financial condition, and accounting are critical to the success of the organization. Since the CNC is an entrepreneurial organization, the importance of teaching entrepreneuring among faculty and students had to be considered. Understanding these processes and how they would serve the CNC administration, practicing faculty, students, and researchers is critical to the selection of supporting software.

Several criteria were used to select off-the-shelf productivity software. Many of these criteria are based on school of nursing corporate decision making to integrate with the executive information system that is concurrently being implemented on a school-wide basis. The criteria are:

1. A commonly known Windows-based user interface;

2. Manufactured by a solid company producing industry standard software with broadly recognized leadership;

3. Integration with other needed software processes, such as word processing;

4. High performance/price ratio;

5. Ease of use;

6. A common macro or scripting language (programming language which would reduce training time for support of the information systems); and

7. Good documentation.

Finally, as mentioned before, effective integration with the second author's development of a school of nursing Executive Information System that will provide executive-level information on the CNC and other strategic plan goals.

The selection of business planning software was a very important decision. Business planning software assists the user in writing a business plan and integrates word processing, spreadsheet, presentation graphics, and project management processes. This software had to be user-friendly for practice faculty who were not familiar with the business planning process, and also adaptable to use in the classroom for educational purposes. Additionally, the CNC administrator would use this software to determine viability of other projects that would have to be evaluated to determine whether they were financially right for the CNC.

Faculty members interested in community-centered practice would need to identify reimbursement methods for generating the portion of their salary devoted to faculty practice. Frequently, this involved development and marketing of a new nursing service in the community. Also, nursing administration students in the financial management course were taught business planning processes and consistent with goals to increase informatics in the curriculum, there was an opportunity to use the business-related software selected for the CNC in the education programming. The business planning software selected was PFS: Business Planner. It was chosen for its strengths in the above-mentioned areas. This software guides the student/faculty through the business planning process. A prepared spreadsheet already has the formulas established that capture unit costs, personnel costs, and transfer these into meaningful information needed to prepare a business plan. An executive summary, graphs that show projections, and a professional business plan is the product of this software package.

Most nursing executives would recognize the need for some type of spreadsheet software package for budgeting and financial management purposes. The business function analysis showed that the *Financial Management* and *Develop Entrepreneurs* functions and some of their associated processes required the use of a spreadsheet software package (see Figure 3). Although there are many acceptable programs on the market, the CNC chose Microsoft Excel for Windows. The school of nursing, the CNC's parent organization, also used this program. Subsequent to that choice, the CNC re-evaluated its need for a separate spreadsheet to meet the information systems' needs of the function of Develop Entrepreneurs. The CNC found that PFS: Business Planner contained an integrated spreadsheet and word processor that behaved substantially like the separate spreadsheet software packages, Microsoft Excel and Word. Consequently, the CNC specified that PFS: Business Planner would be used to support the entrepreneurial function.

Human resource scheduling and project management can break the back of the best staff, so the need to provide software support of this process was identified early (see Figure 2). The above-mentioned criteria were used to select software to support these functions with one exception, there was no need to integrate scheduling data into the executive information system. To allow the CNC to perform administrative human resource scheduling, Microsoft Schedule was chosen to track manager, practitioner, and staff activities.

To perform project management processes, Microsoft Project was selected. This need was assessed with the realization that a separate human resource scheduling system normally used to track individual faculty member's work schedule, such as Microsoft Schedule was not an appropriate decision due to a lack of integration between industry standard business schedulers and clinical practice software.

Additional software was required to complete the support for administrative functions in the CNC. To perform the administrative processes of word processing, communications, and presentation graphics, Microsoft Word, Microsoft Mail, and Microsoft Powerpoint, were chosen (see Figure 2). Scheduling of clients for clinical practice was not considered as a factor when making decisions about administrative scheduling software. Clinical practice software that is available off-the-shelf normally includes a client scheduling module as a natural extension of the electronic client record. The selection of software to support practice and research functions will be discussed in the next section of this chapter.

SUPPORT FOR THE PRACTICE, RESEARCH AND EDUCATION FUNCTIONS

The last three critical success factors dealt with the practice, research, and education functions of the organization. Because one of the CNC's goals and major functions is to accomplish practice-based research, exceptional care should be applied during the information systems planning stage of development. Many of the clinical office practice software packages available off-the-shelf will not provide an adequate database for research purposes.

Most clinical management packages will not support longitudinal analysis of selected variables. The reasons for this are not usually apparent unless you are familiar with *entity modeling* which uses *entity-relationship diagrams* to describe relationships among data entities. Martin (1990a) defines four terms that you need to understand before proceeding—entity, entity model, entity relationship diagram, and data structure. "Entity: A person, place, thing or concept that has characteristics of interest to the enterprise. An entity is something about which we store data" (Martin, 1990a, p. 461). Entities are important to research because they represent exactly what is being studied and enable the researcher to analyze them statistically. The better entities are described and represented, the more suitable the data will be for analysis.

An "Entity Model is a model of the entity types . . . and the relationship between entity types that represent the kind of information needed. . . ." (Martin, 1990a, p. 462). An example of an entity model would be the relationship of the patient identifier (name or unique identification number) to demographic data elements such as age, ethnicity, address, income, blood pressure, and other clinical indicators. An "Entity-Relationship Diagram is a diagram representing entity types and the relationships between them, and certain properties of the relationship . . ." (Martin, 1990a, p. 462).

The concept of data entity relationship is all-important to the researcher. However, it is critical to consider what is happening to the client (patient identifier) and how this type of data needs to be collected on a longitudinal basis. Without the consideration of longitudinality and the follow-on relationships of important entities, there is a strong possibility that some of the needed historical data will not be available for analysis at the end of the data gathering period. For example, a client who visits a neighborhood center may be unemployed, homeless, lack a high school diploma, and be experiencing symptoms of malnutrition and stress. The first demographic data entry will record no income, perhaps no home address, and no high school education when the client is first seen at the center. Over time, as a result of the interventions made by the care providers, the client attains a GED, is assisted to find employment, and has been assisted to find stable housing. If the clinical information system is not designed for longitudinal tracking of demographic data elements such as these, when a change is made in the electronic record to update the client status, the history and consequently tracking of improved outcomes is lost.

Once the software analyst has gathered enough information about the practice and research information needs to create entity relationship diagrams, the analyst can soon create the data structures that will actually contain the data (age, ethnicity, etc.) describing the entity (the patient). Data structures are "a designed and defined collection of record types, linkages, fields . . ." (Martin, 1990a, p. 358).

A data structure contains, at a minimum, fieldnames, field data types, and field lengths. For example, a data structure that will contain client demographic information of last name, first name, and address may contain the following arbitrary field names: LASTNAME, FIRSTNAME, ADDRESSLINEONE, ADDRESSLINETWO, CITY, STATE, ZIP, and INCOME. With the exception of the income field which will be a numeric field, all of the other data types will be character fields, which means that any character, or number, respectively, will be allowed to be stored within the field. The fields will have certain lengths associated with them ranging in this example from 7 to 35 characters or numbers, depending on which field. This simply means that the system will not allow more than the specified number of characters or numbers to be entered into the particular field.

Consequently, after the above data structure has been designed to contain client demographic data, the clinician and/ or the researcher begins to enter data. The following example amplifies the technical information presented previously. The first day that the client presents, she reports that her income is $15,000, so the data entry clerk enters the correct amount into the correct field on her computer screen and the practitioner treats the client. Two years later, during the middle of the researcher's project, the same client returns for additional treatment. A data entry clerk again does her job, entering the client's new annual income of $20,000 into the correct field on the correct screen of her computer. However, if the data structure is not designed for longitudinal data retention, that entry will destroy the original record of the $15,000 annual income data. Due to the absence of the software analyst's consideration of the longitudinal or historical value of the data entity called income, an appropriate data structure was not created to store that data. The result is that the researcher would not be able to test hypotheses related to the socioeconomic variable of income.

From a structured relational database management perspective, for every entity of historical interest that may contain more than one instance of change over time, a data structure dedicated to that entity of interest is required. Otherwise, that entity's history will not be stored beyond each original entry. During the process of software design and development, the software developer should determine which pieces of data (entities) are needed for what purpose and whether a history of changes is required. The software analyst would produce an entity relationship diagram to describe what happens to the data and how they relate to other data. In the case of clinical practice software that will be used for data analysis to support research, the software designer must include a requirement to maintain a history of change of the researcher's variables of interest which could be all or some of the software's data entities. Attention to this requirement will enable the researcher to maintain longitudinal data on changes to variables that are important to his or her research design.

If this longitudinal data management requirement was not considered when the information system was developed, analysis on data entities in clinical datasets and the success of practice-based research is doubtful. If the software designer does not include a research-oriented consideration for one of the data entities for the client's socioeconomic status (such as that described previously in the example related to client income), then the software developer will not create a data table for that data entity. No date-related history of change on the client's socioeconomic status will be maintained and the researcher will not be able to show effects related to that variable.

The only way for CNC administrators to be sure that the data will be available when it is needed is to ask the seller to demonstrate this aspect before purchase of clinical practice software. This requires that CNC administrators and practice and research faculty must know before purchasing clinical practice software which data elements will be important for practice-based research analysis.

Clinical practice software has been discussed from a broad development perspective in the earlier sections of this chapter. Generally, CNCs are faced with two choices, (1) buy off-the-shelf software that was designed with a medical model in mind and possibly without longitudinal considerations of research; or (2) develop from scratch. While the first choice may be practical and may meet the immediate need of getting reimbursed, it may not provide the kind of data that is needed to affect national health policy through research.

The second choice is a lengthy, time-consuming, and usually very costly effort. Assuming that the nurse visionary, and the software designer, analyst, and developer each do their respective parts well, the product will provide lasting service to the clinical practice and research needs. The big health care software companies that manufacture hospital-based products apparently do not yet see a viable CNC market. They will not be willing to spend money developing a nurse-modeled CNC product until they are convinced that the market can afford to purchase the product.

The education function within the CNC is multifaceted. This currently includes educational opportunities for nurse practitioner students, nursing administration students, community health students at the graduate level, small groups of undergraduate students, and a few doctoral students. The planning for information systems is of major importance to student education. It is anticipated that students will participate in learning about the administrative, financial, clinical practice, and research functions of the CNC in the future. This will require time for orientation of students to the software packages used to manage clinical practice and research, and also the selective data related to administrative and financial management. The student education columns on both Figures 4 and 5 reflect the commitment of the CNC to facilitate students' access to CNC information systems. Opportunities to enter and change data will depend on the situation, site, purpose of the data, and in some cases, level of education for the student.

Figure 4   CNC integrated information interrelationships.

C = Creates   U = Uses

Participant(s) / Financial & Entrepreneurial Functions	Client	CEO	Clerical & Billing Staff	Faculty R	Faculty P	Faculty Develop. (Education)	Student Education (Education)
Managing Finances	C	C			U	U	U
Planning Business	C	U			C	C/U	C/U
Supporting Decisions	C/U		C/U	C/U	C/U	C/U	C/U
Administering							
Word Processing	C/U	C/U	C/U	C/U	C/U	C/U	C/U
Presenting	C/U	C/U	C/U	C/U	C/U	C/U	C/U
Scheduling	C/U	C/U	C/U	C/U	C/U	U	U

Figure 5   CNC integrated information interrelationships.

C = Creates   U = Uses

Practice/ Research Functions \ User(s)	Client	CEO	Clerical & Billing Staff	Faculty R	Faculty P	Faculty Develop. (Education)	Student Education
Recording Patient Data	U		C/U	C/U	C/U	U	U
Integrating Practice Data & Costs for Research		C/U		C/U	C/U	C/U	C/U
Calculating Statictics				C/U			C/U
Supporting Decisions	C/U	C/U		C/U			C/U

OVERVIEW MODELING

McFadden and Hoffer (1991, p. 141) as well as Martin (1990a, p. 38) suggest the development of models of the organization which show its components, its organization chart, the flow of information, and the information needed by managers and employees. The products of this phase of the information strategy planning process serve to describe *who* needs what data *when* and for *what* purpose.

Examples of one type of overview modeling is found in Figures 4 and 5, CNC Integrated Information Interrelationships. The left side of both figures contains CNC business functions and respective processes previously discussed and represented in Figures 1, 2, and 3. Again, for this CNC the functions include *education, practice,* and *research* in addition to the functions related to *administration* and *financial management.* In

Figures 4 and 5, the column headings across the top identify the CNC participants involved in these respective business functions and/or processes, such as *faculty, students, CNC CEO, CNC staff,* and so on.

The intersecting cells (identifying who will participate in what function) contain the *type of interaction* that the participant has with the data. In these figures, *"Creates or Uses"* refers to whether the specific person can actually create and/or edit data in the information system or merely view/ use data that someone else has created, possibly for different purposes.

Figures 4 and 5 provide the systems analyst with a functional overview of who needs what data for what purpose in order to carry out the responsibilities of their position in the organization. Information such as this is valuable to the systems analyst from both hardware architecture and software specification perspectives. For example, by studying information from Figures 4 and 5, the analyst would conclude that creators and/or users of the same sets of data would be located in different parts of the same building at best and in different counties at worst. This type of information for an analyst, forms the groundwork for follow-on, in-depth analysis on telecommunications, local area networking (LAN), or even wide area networking (WAN) architectures.

There is important information for the analyst even where there are blanks on tables such as this. The lack of a need to either create or use data can serve as a starting point for decisions regarding access control via password systems, that is, who should be allowed access to what data?

For CNC administrators attempting to initiate the information strategy planning process, Figure 4 shows the results of analyzing the administrative, financial, and entrepreneurial functions of the CNC. Data entry for the majority of these functions is entered by the CNC administrator CEO), administrative assistant, and/or the clerical staff. When Expert Choice is used for corporate level decision making, then faculty and students would be able to enter data. Also, other administrative functions and software would be open for both "creating and using" by all members involved in the CNC.

Some of the financial data used to support the administrative functions within the CNC can only be entered in the CNC office or with clerical staff specifically trained to use the software. This is shown in Figure 4 where faculty and students are only allowed to "use" the financial data. Students and faculty both will have access and be able to "create" or enter data when using the business planning software which involves the business planning function.

The results of analyzing the Practice/Research Functions are shown in Figure 5. One example is the function called Recording Patient Data. Although this table does not show the chronology of the data flow/collection, this aspect was specifically analyzed. On the day that the client presents, the clerical staff receptionist greets the new client and records pertinent data into the clinical practice software system. The receptionist is said to have created the client's record and entered demographics.

Assuming a network is available in this example, upon meeting the new client, the practicing faculty member has available on his or her workstation to the information that was just recorded by the receptionist. Additionally, the practitioner may enter assessment and treatment data into the same system. In this sense, the practitioner has used the receptionist's data and has created clinical data records. Later, the billing staff uses the data created by the receptionist and practitioner to bill the client.

Another important aspect of this process is that faculty researchers can "use" data that both the receptionist and the practitioner have "created" to perform in-depth longitudinal analyses. Researchers also "create" statistical analysis records, and with client confidentiality provisions in place, all of the data is useable in the classroom by the faculty and students. Consequently, note that in the last column under student education, students can both "create and use" data.

For educational purposes, students might be assigned to manipulate data using statistical packages for a project in a graduate or undergraduate research course. Also, doctoral students who may be working on research projects with faculty members may enter actual research data and analyze this data as well. In the area of supporting decisions, graduate or doctoral students using decision analysis software such as Small Tree and/or Expert Choice might enter data as well as use data for educational projects.

There may be some limitations about the ability to enter and change data. Since some of the data entered in the practice arena will be used for research, students may not always be allowed to enter the data. See last column marked education in Figure 5, which limits faculty who are learning the systems (faculty development) and students from entering or changing patient data.

SOFTWARE INTEGRATION

Two of the software selection criteria mentioned relate to integration—the software package's capability to export and import data from and to other specialized software packages. Much of the data that is used in some of the selected software packages is needed by some of the other packages to perform different and more specialized data manipulations. This data exchange, or the ability for one software package to export selected data, and for the receiving software to be able to import that same data for different purposes is important. It is important to do this exporting/importing because no one software package is able to perform all of the processes needed to support a CNC. Figures 6 and 7 indicate the general flow of data among these packages.

For example, on Figure 6 the Electronic Patient Record software package shows cost and billing data and primary care results being collected and exported to a "Research Integrator." The "Research Integrator" is intended to import, integrate, and correlate data exported from other sources. The resultant data are analyzed by statistical software packages such as SPSS for Windows and, in turn, those analytical results are envisioned

Figure 6   Practice/research/education DSS.

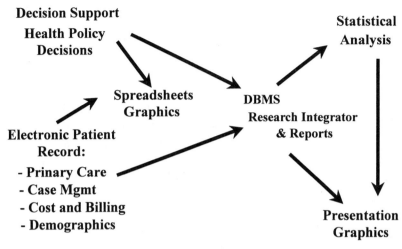

Figure 7   Admin/financial/entrepreneurial DSS.

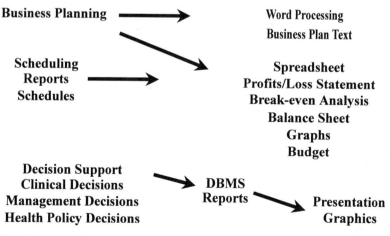

to be exported into presentation graphics software (Microsoft Powerpoint) for presentation and publication to funding agencies and peer groups.

In Figure 7, administrators and entrepreneuring faculty members may create business planning proposals for consideration by other agencies. The results of that planning are integrated within several classes of software, including word processing that contains the narrative of the proposal; a spreadsheet which shows profit/loss, break-even analysis, a budget and a balance sheet; and presentation graphics. Additionally, Figure 7 shows a Database Management System (DBMS) collecting and organizing data from decision support and clinical, management, and health policy decisions. Data from these sources are organized into summary reports and the results of these reports are made available to presentation graphics software for communication.

CONCLUSION

Toffler (1990, p. 163) identifies characteristics of "flex-firm" organizations which are futuristic and have the greatest potential to survive in the future. These organizations will encourage diversity of organizational arrangements with functions and products overlapping. They will be counter bureaucratic in nature and foster networking among groups and departments. Additionally, they will draw information and resources from each other and will be able to trade ideas, data, and strategies efficiently. The University of Rochester CNC can be described in this way. Figure 8 reflects the overlapping of functions and products and proposes counter bureaucratic ways of functioning.

It is not surprising that the information strategy planning process would reflect the overlapping functions and opportunities for administrators, faculty, and students to create and use data and information. For example, data that will be collected

Figure 8 Schematic of the CNC.

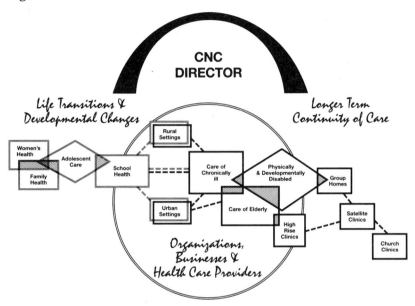

Patricia Hinton Walker, University of Rochester, 1991.

for practice will also be used for research and education functions. Data collected for financial reasons (planning, billing, revenue generating, tracking costs) will also be used for research and education. However, it is very important that CNC administrators clearly identify functions, processes, and critical success factors at the onset of their plan to develop information systems. There will be challenges ahead for all directors of nursing centers as they struggle with the specific challenge of developing information systems support for practice-based research. Information systems development is the key to future survival because they address cost and quality outcomes of nurse-managed care.

REFERENCES

McFadden, F. R., & Hoffer, J. A. (1991). *Database management.* 3rd ed. Redwood City, CA: The Benjamin/Cummings Publishing Company, Inc.

Martin, J. (1990a). *Information engineering book II: Planning and analysis.* Englewood Cliffs, NJ: Prentice Hall.

Martin, J. (1990b). *Information engineering book III: Design and construction.* Englewood Cliffs, NJ: Prentice Hall.

Microsoft Corporation, 1 Microsoft Way, Redmond, WA. (Software)

Potash, M., & Taylor, D. (1993). *Nursing faculty practice: Models and methods.* National Organization of Nurse Practitioner Faculties.

Toffler, A. (1990). *Power shift* (p. 163). New York: Bantam.

Umbaugh, R. E. (ed.). (1991). *Handbook of information systems management.* 3rd ed. Boston, MA: Auerbach.

Walker, P. H. (1991). The community nursing center: For nurse practitioners, an opportunity to develop entrepreneurial skills. *Rochester Nursing,* Fall, 18–19.

6

The Nursing Health Center: A Model of Public/Private Partnership for Health Care Delivery

Kimberly Adams-Davis
Joyce J. Fitzpatrick

Nothing will ever be attempted if all possible obstacles
must first be overcome

Anonymous

*C*urrently there are 250 nursing centers operating in the United States (American Journal of Nursing, 1992). The terms *nurse-managed center, community nursing center/organization,* or *nurse-run clinic* are often used interchangeably. Dominant among definitions, however, is "nurse control of practice and patient care" (Riesch, 1992). In this chapter, we will describe the planning and development of one such community-based nursing center designed to increase access to primary health care services for three inner city urban communities. The Nursing Health Center (NHC) is unique among nursing centers, combining primary health care services for all age groups with the provision of free-standing birthing services for low-risk women. The Frances Payne Bolton School of Nursing of Case Western Reserve University has developed the NHC in collaboration with the City of Cleveland Department of Public Health, Saint Luke's Medical Center, and Metro-Health System of Cuyahoga County.

BACKGROUND

The Frances Payne Bolton School of Nursing has a strong history of aiding underserved populations locally, nationally, and internationally. In 1984, it became apparent to faculty that students educated as certified nurse midwives (CNMs) were not able to fully put into practice the concepts they were taught. The "acute care orientation" of most of the Cleveland area maternity units did not allow for the integration of many midwifery philosophies. Ultimately, in 1991, the closure of Metro-Health Hospital for Women left Cleveland-area women without birthing options.

The School of Nursing faculty saw the need to fill this gap. In October 1991, the School of Nursing responded to the Robert Wood Johnson Foundation, "Local Initiative Funding Partners Program," call for proposals. Stimulated by this opportunity, key health and human service leaders of Greater Cleveland reached a consensus as to the merit of demonstrating such a community-based model of care delivery in this city, and the School of Nursing proceeded with plans for establishing the health center.

Community Assessment

In preparation for submission of the grant proposal, the School of Nursing faculty began an in-depth community assessment. Initially, statistics were gathered from the Federation for Community Planning, the Children's Defense Fund, the Cleveland Center for Economic Development, and the Cleveland Healthy Family/Healthy Start project. After studying these statistics, "windshield tours" of the proposed service areas were conducted in March 1992. These tours provided information about the geographic boundaries of the proposed services area, service providers such as day care centers, grocery stores, churches, schools, health care providers, availability of building space, and general living conditions. Several community development agencies were identified and assistance was sought in locating an appropriate facility. An area councilman also assisted by mailing a needs survey to his constituency. Contact with the Alzheimer's Association revealed that 463 persons living in Mt. Pleasant (population approximately 30,000) had been diagnosed with Alzheimer's disease. Discussions with other community service providers revealed much concern about the vast needs of the elderly populations of the Mt. Pleasant and Buckeye-Shaker communities. The Center for Urban Poverty and Social Change of the Mandel School of Applied Social Sciences, Case Western Reserve University, provided cause of death data for the target communities. This information correlated with City of Cleveland statistics showing *heart disease* and *cancer* as the primary cause of death. As a result of this community assessment, it became apparent that the health care needs of the targeted communities went far beyond needs for maternal-child health care only.

Funding

In December 1992, a proposal was submitted to the Robert Wood Johnson (RWJ) foundation detailing the School of Nursing plans for a full-scope primary health care service managed by advanced practice nurses in collaboration with community residents. As evidence of the developing private/public partnership, the proposal was accompanied by letters of support from state legislators, local private foundations, community residents, the Board of County Commissioners, many service providers, as well as the Mayor of Cleveland. In April 1993, when RWJ staff made a site visit, the depth of the community support and collaboration was demonstrated by the participation of local physicians, a County Commissioner, residents of the target communities, community development agencies, and the NHC collaborating partners.

In June 1993, funding was awarded from the Robert Wood Johnson Foundation. This funding was matched and then exceeded by a local coalition of public and private funders ("The Local Partners"). This funding provided the major portion of startup costs for the support of Center programming. Additional funding was raised for renovation of the NHC facility as a result of the strength of this funding partnership.

NURSING HEALTH CENTER

The NHC is a model of a successful private/public partnership for health care delivery in an era of health care reform. The NHC approach to the delivery of primary health care is three-pronged, providing for traditional clinical services, community outreach activities, and community education programs. Receiving health care services across the life span, residents are encouraged to become involved in their own health care plans. Through culturally sensitive, personalized care, the self-esteem of clients is being enhanced. Should a client require further services, formal arrangements have been made with area physicians for consultation and referral. The NHC acts as the first link to the health care system, providing direct access to secondary and tertiary services when needed. The NHC public/private partnership is developing significant affiliations and referral networks and contracts with physicians, hospitals, and other health care providers. A primary goal is to improve access to health care for inner city residents of the Mt. Pleasant, Buckeye-Shaker, and Woodland Hills communities in Cleveland, Ohio.

The Service Communities

Mt. Pleasant, Buckeye-Shaker, and Woodland Hills are contiguous communities located in an inner-urban area of metropolitan Cleveland within Cuyahoga County. All three areas are comprised of small businesses and residential neighborhoods which have experienced extensive economic and physical decline during the 1970s and 1980s. The majority of buildings are two-family dwellings, many in a state of disrepair. Dispersed among the neighborhoods are numerous churches of a variety of religious denominations. Other neighborhood supports include schools, one senior center, one hospital, and a number of dental offices/clinics. Murtis H. Taylor Multi-Services Center is located near the southeastern border of Mt. Pleasant. While this facility provides some primary health care services, it is at operating capacity, with a general service focus on mental health. Health Hill Hospital, a pediatric rehabilitation facility, is located in Woodland Hills. Located centrally to all three areas is St. Luke's Medical Center. St. Luke's is a source for acute care services in the area and is the primary recipient of NHC referrals.

According to 1990 Census Data, there are a total of 53,471 people living in Mt. Pleasant, Buckeye-Shaker, and Woodland Hills; of these, 18 percent are over the age of 60, and 30 percent are under age 19 (Figure 1). Ninety-three percent of the population is composed of minority groups, primarily African-Americans. The median household income of the

Figure 1 Population by age: 1990 average for target communities.

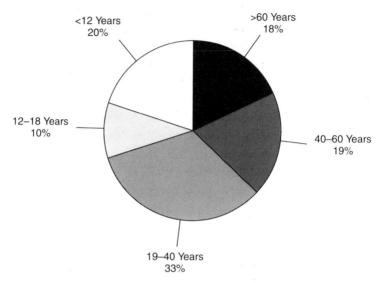

Total Community Population = 53,471

three neighborhoods is $11,604 per year. Thirty-four percent of the people in this community are living at or below the poverty line. Twenty-four percent of households are receiving some form of public assistance (G.A., AFDC, Food Stamps, etc.). Half the family households are headed by females, and the unemployment rate is currently at 12.2 percent (Cleveland Vital Statistics, 1990; Council for Economic Opportunities in Greater Cleveland).

Six of the eleven census tracts in the NHC service areas are federally designated as Medically Underserved or Health Professional Shortage areas. This is reflected in the perinatal data for the targeted neighborhoods based on statistics collected for the period 1988–1990. In these years, the three areas combined had infant mortality rates up to 140 percent (greater than the national average of 10 infant deaths/1,000 live births). In 1990, the average infant mortality rate for the combined area was 24.1 infant deaths/1,000 live births. Two of the neighborhoods, Woodland Hills and Mt. Pleasant, have infant mortality rates of 28.9/1,000 and 26.8/1,000 respectively (Figure 2). Of particular impact on health care costs, with long-term educational and social ramifications, is the high incidence of low birth weight babies. From 1988 through 1990, over 15.2 percent of babies born in the target community fell into this category, a number greater than twice the 1988 U.S. average of 6.9 percent (Figure 3) (Coulton & Chow, 1991). Low birth weight is often the result of inadequate prenatal care, defined as mothers attending fewer than seven prenatal visits (Institute of Medicine, 1985). Within the three social planning areas as well, only 72 percent of pregnant women received adequate prenatal care in 1990 (Figure 4) (Coulton & Chow, 1991); this compares poorly to the U.S. Surgeon General's goal of 90 percent. In addition, 22.9 percent of resident

Figure 2   Infant mortality rate.

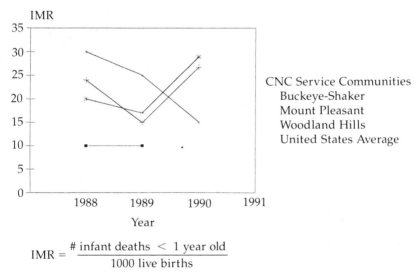

$$IMR = \frac{\text{\# infant deaths} < 1 \text{ year old}}{1000 \text{ live births}}$$

Data from Children's Defense Fund and City of Cleveland/U.S. Vital Statistics.
* Data not available

Figure 3   Low birth weight.

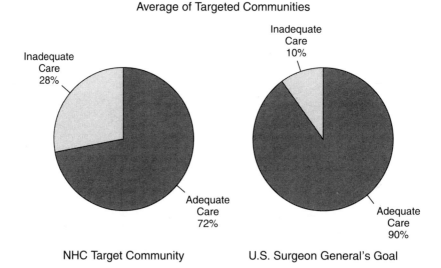

LBW%

25

20

15

10

5

0

1988   1989   1990   1991

Year

Community
  Buckeye-Shaker
  Mount Pleasant
  Woodland Hills
  United States Average

LBW% = Percent of infants born at low birth weight within the area to be served by

Data from Children's Defense Fund and City of Cleveland/U.S. Vital Statistics.
* 1990 Data not available

Figure 4   Inadequate prenatal care (less than 7 visits).

Average of Targeted Communities

Inadequate
Care
28%

Adequate
Care
72%

Inadequate
Care
10%

Adequate
Care
90%

NHC Target Community   U.S. Surgeon General's Goal

teenagers gave birth in 1990, contributing to the high number of low birth weight and premature infants (Coulton & Chow 1991).

ISSUES RELATED TO PRACTICE

Regulatory Issues

During the initial planning, questions arose about the need for the Nursing Health Center to apply for a Certificate of Need (CON) from the Ohio Department of Public Health (ODPH) before initiating birthing service. Inquires to the local Health Systems Agency (HSA) and ODPH resulted in the knowledge that CON approval would be needed. This proved to be a lengthy and expensive process. In the state of Ohio the CON process entails four distinct phases: (1) obtaining an official Determination of Reviewability from the Director of ODPH, (2) submission of the application to the local HSA and the ODPH, (3) submitting formal answers to questions raised by the HSA and the ODPH, and (4) testimony at the Project Review Committee and Board hearings of the HSA. State approval of the CON for birthing facilities was granted May 3, 1994, some 21 months after the process was begun, and as the culmination of a county-wide effort. It is anticipated that renovation of the birthing suites will be completed during September 1994 and birthing services will begin in the fall of 1994.

Many barriers to advanced practice nurses (APNs) providing primary health care existed in the State of Ohio, including: no title recognition for APNs, lack of provisions for direct reimbursement, no prescriptive authority, and the presence and strength of a strong physician lobby. Dealing with these barriers was an essential component to the long-term success of the nurse-managed center. In September 1991, faculty members began visiting legislators to educate them about APN scope of practice and record of service. This strategy was as important as the active participation of the Ohio Nursing Association in the legislative process. Such "visits" were instrumental to the passage of State legislation in December of 1992 to grant the School of Nursing pilot demonstration status. Included in this legislation was a grant to APNs affiliated with the NHC for title recognition, direct reimbursement of medicaid funds, and limited prescriptive authority. Unfortunately, full implementation of the legislation has been impeded by the rule making process and has yet to conclude.

During June 1993, Governor Voinovich approved emergency rules for title recognition. Since that time all eligible NHC nurses have applied to the Ohio Board of Nursing and have been granted recognition as advanced practice nurses. Currently six state-approved advanced practice nurses are employed by the CWRU pilot program. This has led to a stronger movement to extend title recognition to all advanced practice nurses in the state of Ohio.

Emergency rules and regulations for medicaid reimbursement were approved March 1, 1994. The NHC staff has applied for an organizational provider number as well as for individual provider numbers for the Advanced Practice Nurses. The Ohio Department of Human Services has projected that the provider numbers will be granted after July 1994. The Ohio Department of Human Services has made provisions for retroactive billing and reimbursement of services. The NHC and the NHC advanced practice nurses were assigned Medicaid provider numbers during the third week of July.

Prescription Authority

Although all eligible NHC advanced practice nurses have completed the advanced pharmacology course and have met the other requirements, there has not been any implementation of prescriptive authority privileges to date. In addition, a full year passed before the State Medical Board appointed the three physicians to the state-mandated Formulary Committee. In May 1994, 17 months after the passage of the state legislation, emergency rules and regulations were filed by the state mandated Formulary Committee and Governor Voinovich approved the rules. The Formulary Committee proposed changes in these rules and refiled these changes as regular rules in June 1994. The Formulary will then review the pilot program prescriptive authority protocols before approving them in September. Of course, these delays have great potential for limiting the demonstration of the CWRU pilot project, thus restricting access to primary health care services for residents of the Buckeye-Shaker, Mt. Pleasant, and Woodland Hills communities. NHC staff and NHC consulting physicians have developed a plan to bridge this gap during this interim period. At present, NHC staff is working with Board of Nursing staff and the Formulary Committee to negotiate prescriptive authority protocols and to establish a firm timetable for the implementation of prescriptive authority for NHC advanced practice nurse. It is anticipated that the rules and regulations for prescriptive authority will be approved in October.

Insurance

During the planning for the NHC, it became apparent that adequate insurance coverage for professional and commercial needs would be essential to successful operations. The acquisition of organizational malpractice insurance for the NHC was a tedious and lengthy process. NHC staff began to make formal inquiries regarding malpractice insurance in March 1992. Multiple discussions and submission of applications resulted in premium quotes that ranged from $75,000 to $125,000, annually. The insurance companies stated that the NHC was considered to be "a risk" because nurse-control of clinical practice is uncommon. This experience led NHC staff to the realization that education of insurance brokers and underwriters about the history of advanced practice nurses, particularly nurse-midwives, quality of care, and the history of malpractice related to APN service would be important to obtaining affordable and adequate coverage. It was also important for NHC staff to become familiar with insurance industry terminology and norms. Over the next 10–14 months, NHC staff submitted numerous applications and application revisions to insurance underwriters via a major insurance broker. In April 1994, malpractice insurance was finally purchased for a fee of $26,000. NHC advanced practice nurses are also individually insured for malpractice.

The acquisition of director and officers insurance followed a similar pattern. After many months of preparation, a final quote for director and officers insurance was only obtained after NHC staff personally answered the concerns of the underwriter in a hour-long telephone call.

Staffing

The NHC assures continuity and quality of care through its staffing structure. The director of the NHC heads a staff of advanced practice nurses. The nursing staff includes an Ob-Gyn nurse practitioner, a certified nurse-midwife, a pediatric nurse practitioner, adult nurse practitioner, and public health nurse. Community Health Advocates recruited from area residents aid the nurses in all aspects of primary care delivery, and help the nurses identify and approach residents who could benefit from services. In general, NHC staff have found that true public/private partnerships are key to successful service provision.

In the effort to secure public/private partnerships, support staff plays a significant role. Support staff includes a full-time business manager, an administrative assistant, contractual maintenance and housekeeping personnel, and physician consultants.

CURRENT OPERATIONS

During the past 10 months, the NHC staff has focused on building community support and awareness of NHC services through intensive community outreach and educational programs. NHC staff have participated in numerous community activities, such as providing screening services at local churches, working with local schools to enhance health education for children, distribution of health education materials through street canvasing, and hosting community open houses with other service agencies. The opening of the Buckeye Road facility on May 17, 1994, enabled the staff to supplement these services with traditional services (prenatal care, physical examinations, and facility-based education programming etc). Initial clientele have included clients from the target service area, clients from other communities, as well as School of Nursing faculty and students.

FUTURE PLANS

Plans for the next year of operations include (1) the development of a comprehensive plan for communications, (2) the cultivation of a stronger community presence through continued community outreach and collaboration with other agencies, (3) the continued refinement of practice and policy protocols, and (4) the enhancement of the NHC business plan.

CONCLUSION

Collaboration with community residents is paramount to the success of the NHC public/private partnership and ultimately the successful provision of primary health care services. Community resident input regarding service is continually sought through activities such as community focus groups, staff attendance at community meetings, community resident representation on the Board of Trustees, as well the NHC Community Advisory Committee, and other community outreach activities. NHC staff persist in using this input to direct and shape all NHC services.

REFERENCES

American Journal of Nursing. (1992). Community Nursing Centers gaining ground as solution to health issues. *American Journal of Nursing, 92*(7), 70–71.

Coulton, C. J., & Chow, J. (1991). *An analysis of infant mortality in the Cleveland area.* Cleveland, OH: Case Western Reserve University.

Institute of Medicine. (1988). *Preventing low birth weight.* Washington, DC: National Academy Press.

Riesch, S. K. (1992). Nursing centers: An analysis of anecdotal literature. *Journal of Professional Nursing, 8*(1), 16–25.

7

The Family Nursing Center at Gladstone School: A Nursing Model for Primary Health Care

Janice S. Borman
Lorna Finnegan
Mary Oesterle
Susan Swider

The historic mission or purpose of universities, i.e., assist through education with programmes in professional manpower development; advance knowledge through research, both basic and applied; and provide service through constant interaction with the community are all highly suitable for improving the health of populations.

WHO, 1985

*C*onsistent with the World Health Organization's (WHO's) statement that universities' historical missions are suitable for improving the health of populations (WHO, 1989), Saint Xavier University School of Nursing established a partnership with a Chicago public school to provide family-centered primary health care. The product of this partnership is the Family Nursing Center at the William E. Gladstone Elementary School. The Family Nursing Center is designed in the vision of Nursing's Agenda for Health Care Reform in that it is a consumer-driven, community-based system of primary health care (ANA, 1991). It is also a model for integrating primary health care into the curriculum of a school of nursing to help prepare competent practitioners for a revisioned health care system. Faculty practice in the Center will demonstrate integration of the faculty's teaching, practice and research roles within a primary health care setting.

The purpose of this chapter is to describe the overall goals and objectives of the Family Nursing Center in relation to primary health care, and the activities undertaken to implement the Center in its first seven months.

BACKGROUND

Gladstone School is a public elementary school located on the west side of the city of Chicago. The school, one of the oldest in the city, has historically been a stable element in this low-income, African-American community. Many faculty currently teach the children of their former students. The school serves approximately 500 students in grades prekindergarten through eight, as well as various special education programs.

Although the motto of Gladstone School is "The Pride of the West Side," the school faces overwhelming challenges. Demographic characteristics reveal a community at risk of experiencing above average rates of death, disease, and disability. The community is 97 percent African-American, with approximately 50 percent of the families living at or below the poverty level. All the children attending Gladstone School are from low-income families (Gladstone School Report Card, 1992). Statistics reveal that the Gladstone community is experiencing those problems that often affect poor, inner-city, African-American communities, including high rates of homicide, accidents, communicable illness, and sexually transmitted diseases (Masterson, 1994; Young, 1994).

Although Gladstone School is in close proximity to several major medical centers, the Gladstone community is designated a medically underserved community. Residents of the Gladstone Community face multiple barriers in obtaining health care. Many community residents have no health insurance coverage, or are covered under Medicaid, which limits choice of providers. The available providers are often inaccessible in terms of location, hours or cultural sensitivity.

Gladstone School staff have identified and have been long concerned about the significant health issues that affect the school's students. These issues include a lack of immunizations, poor hygiene practices, poor nutrition, and a lack of self-care knowledge. After hearing a Saint Xavier University faculty member present on the role of advanced practice nurses, the principal of the Gladstone School contacted Saint Xavier University nursing faculty to determine if advanced practice nurses could begin to address some of the health issues in the school. As a result of that contact, Saint Xavier University School of Nursing faculty and Gladstone School personnel met to explore ways to work together to address the primary health care needs in the community.

Nursing Education's Needs

Saint Xavier University's mission has long been to serve the educational and social needs of the Chicago area. In this tradition of service, nursing faculty have had a small nurse-managed center on the University's campus since 1986. At this site, nursing care services were delivered to members of the Saint Xavier University community and the community at large. Over time, faculty expressed interest in developing an off-campus nursing center to further their efforts to revise their curriculum to meet the mandates set forth by *Nursing's Agenda for Health Care Reform* (ANA, 1991). Inherent in the *Agenda for Health Care Reform* is a consumer-driven, community-based primary health care system. Consistent with this, both the National League for Nursing (NLN) and the American Association of Colleges of Nursing (AACN) have identified agendas for nursing education reform that include increasing the number of advanced nurse practitioners and reforming educational programs to assure competency in community-based primary health care, health promotion, cost-effective coordinated care, and working with diverse ethnic, minority, and underserved populations (AACN, 1992; NLN, 1992).

Providing direct care services as a means of integrating the teaching, research, and practice missions of schools of nursing is one vehicle through which nursing is beginning to address the need for integration of primary health care content throughout the curriculum (AACN, 1992). Faculty practice serves as a strategy for fostering linkages between schools of nursing and their communities (NLN, 1992). As faculty explore the intricacies of working in extra-institutional sites and focus more on population-based care and collaborative relationships with consumers, they are assuming responsibility for preparing graduates that will be competent in providing community-based care (AACN, 1992). With these goals in mind, the Saint Xavier University nursing faculty worked with the Gladstone community to develop the Family Nursing Center at Gladstone School.

CONCEPTUAL FRAMEWORK

Primary health care, as articulated by WHO, is the underlying philosophy of the Family Nursing Center at Gladstone. Primary health care is defined as essential health care made universally accessible and acceptable to people in a community through their full participation and at cost the community can afford.

In this framework, health is viewed as integrally related to the social and economic development of the community (WHO, 1978). This framework calls upon nurses to work in partnership with communities to improve health within the context of social and economic development.

Igoe and Giordano (1992) view this as a redefinition of nursing roles or a "provider role shift" in which consumers will form partnerships with an "exchange information" with health care providers. As stable community centers, school-based family health care centers are viewed as a viable strategy for facilitating this provider role shift. Nurses will be key players in this plan to return ownership for health and health information to the consumer (Igoe & Giordano, 1992).

Design of a Family Nursing Center

In keeping with the primary health care approach, the Family Nursing Center at Gladstone was designed to have community members and nurses work collaboratively to identify the community's health needs and plan for services. These services then would be provided by Saint Xavier University nursing faculty, students, and community members themselves, as appropriate.

Saint Xavier University was funded by the Department of Health and Human Services, Division of Nursing in September 1993 to implement the Family Nursing Center at Gladstone School. The overall goal of the Center is to demonstrate a nursing model of primary health care. To meet this goal, the Center has four specific objectives:

1. Provide primary health care services with children and families using Gladstone School as the point of entry.
2. Demonstrate primary health care practice by faculty and students in a family nursing center.
3. Empower families to participate in primary health care using referral and advocacy strategies.

4. Evaluate the quality outcomes and cost effectiveness of the Family Nursing Center.

These objectives reflect the key components of primary health care, as well as the need to incorporate primary health care in the nursing curriculum.

Project personnel for the Family Nursing Center include faculty who serve as the program director, the project director/ evaluator, the faculty practice consultant, two family nurse practitioners, the community advocate consultant, and two community health nursing teachers. Other project staff include a community nurse specialist, two community health advocates, an information systems consultant, and a secretary.

The remainder of this chapter will discuss the activities undertaken to implement the center in its first seven months. These activities served to meet multiple project objectives and thus have been grouped according to the functional areas in the first year of the project. These areas include community assessment and collaboration, delivery of primary health care services through a faculty practice model, and evaluation of quality outcomes and cost effectiveness.

IMPLEMENTATION

Community Collaboration and Assessment

Key to the model of primary health care is the importance of working with community residents, from the beginning, to define health concerns and develop, implement and evaluate means to address these concerns. Thus, many of the activities in the first year of development of the Family Nursing Center focused on continuing to work with the Gladstone community to define health needs and begin to plan to address them. This is vital because community residents understand their lives and needs better than health professionals from the outside. In addition, primary health care recognizes that most of what makes people healthy happens in homes and communities. Thus, to enlist community participation in improving their overall health, it is imperative to have the community involved in defining health and determining priorities for action that are consistent with the community's lived experience.

One means of enlisting community collaboration in health improvement efforts has been to bring health care to where people live and work, via training and utilization of community health advocates (CHAs). A WHO study group formed to examine issues relating to the use of CHAs identified CHAs as a means of addressing the limits of traditional medicine in improving health (WHO, 1989). Similar arguments have been made that medical services do not adequately address the social, environmental, and cultural factors that cause disease and disability, but that community-based activities led by CHAs may be more effective (Bender & Pitkin, 1987; Hatch & Eng, 1983; Matemora, 1989; McElmurry et al., 1990; Swider & McElmurry, 1990; WHO, 1989).

The CHA role is a bridge between the community and the health system. There is agreement in the literature that this role has three components: (1) translating the community's concerns to the health care system and vice versa, (2) providing linkages between the community and the health care system, and (3) enabling the community's actions to influence their own health and development (Giblin, 1989; Marquez et al., 1987; Matemora, 1989). However, the role of the CHA also needs to reflect the needs of the community, and allow sufficient flexibility for the CHA to adapt and adopt creative solutions to community health and development problems (WHO, 1978).

CHAs are defined as community residents who receive special training to help bring health services and education to their communities, and mobilize the community for action to improve health and living conditions. CHAs thus work closely with both community residents and with health care professionals. They serve as a bridge between their community and the formal health care system. CHAs have been shown to be most effective in this role when they are selected by and from the community in which they will work, thus enhancing their acceptance by, and responsibility towards, their neighbors (Bender & Pitkin, 1987; Matemora, 1989; WHO, 1989).

The CHA position requirements for the Family Nursing Center at Gladstone School included a high school diploma or the equivalent, status as a community resident and/or a Gladstone parent, and interest in and/or a history of community involvement (either paid or volunteer). Recommendations for the CHA position were solicited from Gladstone staff and parents.

Interviews for the position were conducted by a team consisting of the community advocate consultant, one of the project's family nurse practitioners, Gladstone's school community representative, and Gladstone's assistant principal. The applicant chosen for the CHA position was a young woman with two children, one of whom attends the school. She is also caring for two nephews, both of whom attend Gladstone School. She is a member of the local school council, has been an active and involved parent volunteer at the school, and has lived in the community for over 20 years.

Training needs of the CHA are related to the need for nontraditional educational methods, training that is relevant to the community's culture and needs, and ongoing continuing education (Soares, Swider, & McElmurry, 1994; Swider & McElmurry, 1990). Thus, one CHA in this project received her initial training in an established training program for CHAs at the University of Illinois at Chicago College of Nursing (Swider & McElmurry, 1990). This training program for CHAs, based on the primary health care approach to community health improvement as articulated by WHO, has been in existence since 1982. The purpose of this training is to develop within trainees basic health knowledge for individuals and communities, basic personal and community development skills, skills for community assessment, and advocacy skills.

In addition, a current school employee who serves as a community liaison for the school has received some training as a CHA to expand her vital role in community outreach to include health-related concerns. These two women teach their neighbors about health in a way that formal health care providers and systems never achieve. Examples of this include health information and teaching that takes place in the evenings or on weekends as part of neighborly communications. In addition, these CHAs can express community needs and strengths from the perspective of their personal experience. They also recruit members for the asthma class and immunization drives, which will be discussed later. They reach parents in their homes to discuss their children's health needs, as well as represent the Family Nursing Center in a variety of community settings such as churches and the local school council.

To further structure opportunities for collaboration with community members, the Family Nursing Center staff developed a community advisory board to help in determining Family Nursing Center program priorities, planning, and methods to reach out to community members. The board includes teachers, students, local service providers, parents, community activists, and community religious leaders. In the first seven months of the project, the advisory board has met three times to discuss community needs. As time passes, further participation of each of these members in outreach and program implementation will be solicited.

Enlisting community participation in health promotion efforts also includes assessing community perceptions of health needs and resources. In the initial year of the Family Nursing Center, formal community assessments were conducted by graduate students, incorporating demographic, morbidity, and mortality data for the community with key informant interviews and windshield surveys. Additionally, project personnel, with the assistance of the CHAs and undergraduate students in community health nursing, have surveyed parents, teachers, the advisory board, and Gladstone students for their perceptions of health needs in the school and community. One CHA has also been developing a directory of community resources in relation to health and development. These resources will help in program planning and improving access to services for the community. In addition, the process of documenting these resources has served to introduce the Family Nursing Center concept and the CHAs to other community agencies, for future collaboration.

Delivery of Primary Health Care Services Through a Faculty Practice Model

Primary health care services through the Family Nursing Center at Gladstone have been provided using a faculty practice model of care delivery. Faculty practice includes all aspects of the delivery of nursing service through the role of clinician, educator, researcher, consultant, and administrator (Potash & Taylor, 1993). The Family Nursing Center provides a mechanism to unify the multiple demands of education, practice, and research, as well as to exercise control and maximize effectiveness of faculty-related activities. Faculty practice is used as a strategy to fashion linkages between Saint Xavier University School of Nursing and the community that is served by Gladstone School. Through faculty practice, faculty who are comfortable with community-based primary health care assist in preparing the practitioners of the future as well as model this type of practice for other faculty who are not yet comfortable with community-based primary health care. Few faculty have been introduced to the future consumer-driven, community-based primary health care system, and even fewer are comfortable with their roles in such a system (NLN, 1992). Thus, the mission of nursing education is increasingly not only to promote quality care by educating qualified practitioners, but to create linkages that allow the educational projects of faculty and students to provide services.

Faculty who teach in community health nursing and those who teach in the Family Nurse Practitioner program surfaced as faculty who are most comfortable with community-based primary health care. Consistent with the faculty practice model, primary health care services have been provided by these faculty along with their students.

Community Health Nursing Faculty Practice. Community health nursing faculty began practicing at Gladstone prior to the inception of funding for the project. During April 1993, community health nursing students and faculty worked collaboratively with the Chicago Department of Health to conduct an immunization campaign at Gladstone School. By the following academic year, 250 children were out of compliance with state immunization requirements as a result of a recent Illinois requirement that all elementary students receive a second measles vaccination before entering school. The undergraduate community health nursing students thus developed and implemented a plan for community outreach and education about the importance of immunizations. During a subsequent one-day event, 140 Gladstone students were immunized. Additional immunization events were held in September and December 1993 and January 1994. By February 1994, Gladstone School had only nine children who were excluded from school for lack of compliance with state health requirements. The school nurse at Gladstone confirmed that, based on her experience, Gladstone School had a much better compliance rate than other Chicago public schools, due in large part to the efforts of the Family Nursing Center.

Additional primary health care services provided by community health nursing faculty and students included conducting classroom teaching activities on health-related topics such as oral hygiene, general hygiene, dental care, handwashing, and nutrition; developing a directory of available health and social services resources for the community for future use as a referral system; and surveying health records. A recent endeavor involved piloting an illness management education program for children with asthma in conjunction with the Chicago Lung Association.

Family Nurse Practitioner Faculty Practice. Family nurse practitioner faculty, along with their students, conducted a screening event that provided the eighth-grade students with the opportunity to receive the physical exams required for high-school entrance. During April 1994, 47 eighth-grade students made "field trips" to the Saint Xavier University campus. During these field trips, the Gladstone students had their physical exams completed by the Family Nurse Practitioner faculty and students. This served as a model of faculty practicing collaboratively with nursing students, as well as a mechanism to deliver these services to the Gladstone students. Multiple health promotion needs as well as some health problems were identified. Some of these Gladstone students will be followed at the Family Nursing Center.

As a part of their field trip, Gladstone students also participated in (1) presentations offered by Saint Xavier University's Admissions Department and (2) focus groups conducted by the community nurse specialist on this project. The Admissions Department, along with a panel of African-American college students, shared strategies for goal-setting with respect to careers, as well as perspectives on how to achieve those goals. During the focus groups, Gladstone students shared their perspectives on their health needs and services they desired at the Family Nursing Center.

Physical Facilities Required for Faculty Practice. Through interorganizational planning between the Chicago Public Schools and Saint Xavier University School of Nursing, a classroom at Gladstone School was renovated to house the Family Nursing Center. The Center includes three examination rooms, a conference room, storage, and office space. This newly renovated space allows family nurse practitioner faculty practice at the Center to meet students' health promotion needs or health problems. Community health and other nursing faculty will also use the facilities with their undergraduate and graduate nursing students.

Integration of Primary Health Care into the Curriculum. In Spring 1994, the faculty practice consultant organized a student-faculty forum on the students' experiences at the Family Nursing Center. The purpose of the forum was to promote understanding among the school of nursing's faculty about the type of student experiences possible in a nurse-managed center, thus stimulating interest in developing further clinical experiences at the Family Nursing Center to allow integration of primary health care into the school of nursing's curriculum. Four undergraduate nursing students presented the projects they undertook at the nursing center, including immunization clinics, an asthma education program, nutrition bingo, and a parent survey. The principal of Gladstone School and Saint Xavier University faculty, staff, and students participated in a discussion of these projects, as well as the promise the Family Nursing Center holds for students across the curriculum of the school of nursing. This is one method used to facilitate integration of primary health care into the school of nursing's curriculum.

An additional method is to have project personnel attend curriculum meetings. The faculty practice consultant on the project attends Undergraduate Curriculum Committee meetings to facilitate the process of expanding primary care concepts and experiences throughout the undergraduate curriculum. Two project team members serve as members of the Graduate Curriculum Committee. These project team members have an opportunity to discuss primary health care concepts and experiences in the context of their committee membership.

Evaluation of Quality Outcomes and Cost Effectiveness

Evaluation goals for the Family Nursing Center involve determining the effectiveness of the primary health care approach for improving the health of the Gladstone community, specifically in the areas of quality and cost effectiveness of primary health care activities. Such an evaluation will assist in determining the replicatibility of this model in other locations. Evaluation additionally serves as an excellent learning experience for nursing students at all levels. Undergraduate students can view evaluation as part of the nursing process at the community level. Graduate students can begin to understand how evaluation is designed and implemented in practice.

A Management Information System. One of the first activities in the evaluation process was to select and implement a management information system (MIS) to track data and investigate relationships among the data. An MIS allows the Family Nursing Center to efficiently manage itself, establish the costs of the primary health care services provided, evaluate its cost effectiveness and quality outcomes, and bill for services. According to Marchello (1991), the MIS must have client database management capabilities; clinic utilization and clinical databases, with database management capabilities; financial database management capabilities; and the ability to generate reports financial, client, and provider information.

Prior to being able to identify a consultant for the implementation of such an information system, it was necessary to identify the information structure of the system. Various medical practice packages were reviewed and rejected because of their inability to capture nursing information and/or the costliness of customizing them to capture nursing information. The Omaha System was identified as a likely taxonomy on which to base the information system. The Omaha System is a well-used system of documenting nursing practice. At this time, many community-based nursing practices nationwide are using the Omaha System. The system, which evolved over 15 years of effort and seven years of federally funded research, consists of a Problem Classification Scheme, and Intervention Scheme, and a Problem Rating of Outcomes (Martin & Scheet, 1992). According to Martin and Scheet (1992), the Omaha System is a structured, comprehensive approach to community health practice, documentation, and data management. Therefore the system offers the following six capabilities and characteristics for community health nursing:

- Advances in scientific practice of nursing
- Capabilities to quantify community health nursing

• Practicality for general community health application
• Congruency with the nursing process
• Minimized redundancy in the client record
• Limited documentation time (p. 20).

A review of the literature and at least 25 contacts were made nationwide to determine who was using the Omaha System and if automated systems were available for purchase. The result of the search indicated that most nursing centers use a nonautomated version of the Omaha System and those who use an automated version are not making their system available to others. Based on this information, The Information System Consultant on the project developed a customized information system. It combines a fully integrated practice management system, named Foxmed Pro, with an automated version of the Omaha System. The practice management database includes customized client demographic and clinical components, customized clinic and provider information components, an accounting package, electronic billing, a patient scheduling module, a report generator, and system security. The entire information system (hardware and software) is at Gladstone School and Saint Xavier University, connected by modem.

The Omaha System is currently designed to capture data at the level of the individual and the family. As project activities will also be directed at the level of the community, community-level data must also be captured for evaluation purposes. Conceptually, the Omaha System is appropriate at the community level, although few have attempted to operationalize it at this level (K. Martin, personal communication, April 12, 1994). During subsequent years of the project, attempts will be made to capture community-level data with the MIS for evaluation purposes.

Quality. Another set of evaluation activities focuses on evaluating the quality of primary health care activities conducted by the Center. There are already established quality measures for clinic services that are being reviewed and revised as appropriate. Work has begun on developing quality indicators as part of developing the Center's policies and procedures. Quality indicators are being developed from the Pace University Nursing Center quality of care standards and various standards for quality set by the American Nurses Association and the National League of Nursing.

The quality of health education and advocacy activities are more difficult to evaluate in terms other than participation rates and client satisfaction. Center staff will focus on documenting such activities via an encounter form, which details the purpose of the activity, the audience and its demographics, the immediate outcome and any follow-up needed. After several years of this documentation, along with computerization of these records, the staff will develop a plan for measuring outcomes of these activities. This might include pre- and post-tests of knowledge changes, focus groups or interviews on behavior changes, and cost-effectiveness measures of referral and advocacy services. It is anticipated that additional outside funding would be sought for support of this research. There are beginning efforts towards such evaluation in the international literature on primary health care and CHAs, and these would serve as a starting point for our efforts (Giblin, 1989; WHO, 1989).

Costs.   Another goal is estimating the costs of the services provided, and evaluating these costs in terms of outcome measures. As such, these activities will rely heavily on the data generated by the MIS system and the outcome measures. This work is vital in arguing for funds to sustain this model and in trying to replicate this service-education approach elsewhere.

As part of evaluating costs, a fee structure is being investigated. It will be dependent on the Medicaid billing structure because such a large percentage of the Gladstone population receives Medicaid benefits. The information system implemented allows for future electronic billing, if appropriate. A sliding fee scale is being developed with the assistance of a financial consultant. A recent Illinois Attorney General's opinion may pave the way for family nurse practitioners to become recognized by the Illinois Department of Public Aid as providers of primary care services and thus receive Medicaid reimbursement.

FUTURE PLANS

The Family Nursing Center's initial focus has been on the school children attending Gladstone School. However, in subsequent years, the Center will expand its focus to include the families of these children and other community residents. This will be accomplished by the expansion of faculty practice in the Center as well as a more comprehensive integration of primary health care concepts across the curriculum.

Faculty and student practice in the Family Nursing Center will be expanded consistent with the Family Nursing Center Advisory Board priorities, as well as community needs as documented in currently available and ongoing assessment data. As clinical experiences are proposed, they will be subject to review by the Family Nursing Center's Advisory Board to assure that they are acceptable and appropriate to the needs of the community. Similarly, any research-related activities will be subject to a Research Review Board that will represent the interests of both the academic and the Gladstone community.

An initial area for expansion of community health nursing student experiences includes significant focus on community outreach, including home visiting. Students will link with Chicago Department of Health nurses to share in case finding and case management for families in the Gladstone community. In addition, community health nursing faculty will be able to carry case loads in the community as part of their own faculty practice.

As senior-level community health nursing students move to a more proficient level of practice, many of the health screening and health education activities in the Family Nursing Center can be assumed by students at junior and sophomore levels. A minimum of at least 25 percent of the nursing students at Saint

Xavier University should have a significant clinical experience at the Family Nursing Center. The current health promotion focus at the lower levels in the curriculum will be enhanced by moving clinical experiences within a nursing practice model. Integration of clinical practice in this community-based site from the very earliest points in the curriculum will reinforce the importance of primary health care and a future-oriented perspective on health care delivery.

In addition to curricular needs of students, faculty practice interests will shape other initiatives within the Family Nursing Center. Faculty from a variety of specialty backgrounds will have the opportunity to define their practices to address the defined and emerging needs of the Gladstone community. As faculty engage in their own practice, they will enhance their own proficiency in delivery of primary health care services, as well as offer an increasingly broad model of nursing practice. The Community Health and Family Nurse Practitioner faculty are currently the first faculty to practice and are providing a prototype, but the opportunities for other faculty prepared as clinical nurse specialists are similarly rich.

The stability of the relationship between the CHAs and those who practice in the Family Nursing Center is pivotal in the growth of services in the Center. The CHAs are seen as central in reflecting the needs of the community and helping to define flexible ways to address those needs. The CHAs will help to shape faculty and student services that will be acceptable to the community. The CHAs will also identify available resources that can be interfaced with services provided in the Family Nursing Center and help initiate community-level efforts toward health improvement. The role of the CHAs will continue to be that of providing an essential linkage between the community, the Family Nursing Center, and the larger health care system.

As faculty move into a variety of practice roles, the opportunities to generate revenue in this nursing model will simultaneously grow. Reimbursement for services provided in the Family Nursing Center is pivotal to long-term sustainability of the Nursing Center. The MIS is essential to the determining the

Center's costs, as well as anticipating revenue from billing. Additionally, the MIS will allow the Family Nursing Center to document the quality of care, the outcomes and the cost effectiveness of this nursing model.

SUMMARY

This chapter described the Family Nursing Center at Gladstone School, which is a nursing model for primary care health care. The development of the model has been presented, emphasizing the underlying tenants of primary health care and the priorities of *Nursing's Agenda for Health Care Reform* (ANA, 1991). The overall goals of the Family Nursing Center and the activities to be undertaken to implement the Center in its first seven months were discussed. Finally, future directions for the Center were defined.

REFERENCES

American Association of Colleges of Nursing. (1992). Position statement for addressing nursing educations agenda for the 21st century. Washington DC: American Association of Colleges of Nursing.

American Nurses Association. (1991). *Nursing's agenda for health care reform*. Washington, DC: Author.

Bender, D. E., & Pitkin, K. (1987). Bridging the gap: The village health worker as the cornerstone of the primary health care model. *Social Science Medicine, 24*, 515–528.

Giblin, P. T. (1989). Effective utilization and evaluation of indigenous health care workers. *Public Health Reports, 104*, 361–368.

Gladstone School Report Card, 1992.

Hatch, J., & Eng, E. (1983). Health workers roles in community oriented primary care. In E. Connor & R. Mallan (Eds.), *Community oriented primary care*. Washington, DC: National Academy Press.

Igoe, J. B., & Giordano, B. P. (1992). *Expanding school health services to serve families in the 21st century*. Washington, DC: American Nurses Publishing.

Illinois Nurses Association. (January, 1994). News Release.

Marchello, M. (Ed.). (1991). *Clinic management information system.* New York: Lienhard School of Nursing, Pace University.

Marquez, L. R., Brownlee, A., Molzan, J., Reynolds, J., & Sums, L. (1987). *Community health workers: A comparative analyses of prior-funded studies.* Chevy Chase, MD: Pricor, Center for Human Services.

Martin, K. (April 12, 1994). Personal communication.

Martin, L., & Scheet, N. (1992). *The Omaha system: Applications for community health nursing.* Philadelphia: Saunders.

Masterson, T. (1994). Community assessment. Unpublished manuscript.

Matemora, M. K. S. (1989). Mass produced village health workers and the promise of primary health care. *Social Science Medicine, 28,* 1081–1084.

McElmurry, B., Swider, S., Bless, C., Murphy, D., Montgomery, A., Norr, K., Irwin, Y., Gantes, M., & Fisher, M. (1990). Community health advocacy: Primary health care nurse-advocate teams in urban communities. In *Perspectives in nursing 1989–1991.* New York: National League for Nursing.

National League for Nursing. (1992). *An agenda for nursing education reform.* New York: National League for Nursing.

Pace University. (1991). *Workbook on establishing at nurse-managed health center.* New York: Lienhard School of Nursing, Pace University.

Potash, M., & Taylor, D. (1993). *Nursing faculty practice: Models and methods.* National Organization for Nurse Practitioner Faculties.

Soares, C., Swider, S., & McElmurry, B. (1994). The training of community health advocates: A program evaluation. Unpublished manuscript.

Swider, S. M., & McElmurry, B. J. (1990). A women's health perspective in primary health care: A nursing and community health worker demonstration project in urban America. *Family Community Health, 13*(3), 1–17.

World Health Organization. (1978). *Primary health care.* Geneva: World Health Organization.

World Health Organization. (1989). *Strengthening the performance of community health workers in primary health care.* Geneva: World Health Organization.

Young, L. (1994). Community Assessment. Unpublished manuscript.

8

Building an Entrepreneurial Multi-Site Autonomous Practice in a Rural Community

Peter Coggiola
Patricia Hinton Walker

The decision to open a nurse practitioner practice is often difficult to make. Success depends on the possession of specific resources, such as adequate skills, finances, emotional support and the desire to be one's own boss.

Calmelat, 1993

*T*he development of autonomous practice roles of nurse practitioners for primary care is an important topic in the nursing literature in the context of health care reform. "Everyone from consumers to policy makers understands the engines that drive our health care systems—access, cost, and quality—are out of control" according to Kraus (1992). The major goal of many of the health care reform plans currently debated on capitol hill is that Americans have affordable, accessible, cost effective, and quality health care. To achieve this goal, one proposed solution to the problem of mal-distribution and cost is the increased utilization of advanced practice nurses to provide primary care, especially in underserved areas.

The nursing literature provides numerous examples of studies supporting the value and quality of care provided by nurse practitioners compared to their physician (MD) colleagues (Bessman, 1974; Brown & Grimes, 1993; Chambers & West, 1978; Charney & Kitzman, 1971; Komaroff, Sawayer, Flatley, & Browne, 1976; Lewis & Resnick, 1967; Lewis, Resnick, Schmidt, & Waxman, 1969; McLaughlin et al., 1979; Scherer, Fortin, Spitzer, & Kergin, 1977; Spitzer et al., 1974). Regardless of the fact that many of these studies have been criticized because of lack of control for severity of illness, results consistently indicated that nurse practitioner care was comparable to technical care provided by physicians (Chen, Barkauskas, Ohlson, Chen, & DeStefano, 1983).

More recently, additional studies have examined the interaction process between health care provider and patient. Results indicated that nurse practitioner's are more successful with history taking, patient understanding, dealing with psychosocial concerns, and facilitating behavioral modifications (Campbell, Mauksch, Heikirk, & Hosokawa, 1990; Goodman & Perrin, 1978; Perrin & Goodman, 1978; Ramsay, McKenzie, & Fish, 1982; Stein, 1972). Avorn, Everitt, and Baker (1991) conducted a study using case vignettes. Results of this study indicated that nurse practitioners were more likely than physicians to inquire about a patient's diet and psychosocial factors. Consequently, nurse practitioners were more likely to prescribe relevant behavioral changes than write prescriptions for costly medications. Safriet (1992), in a significant article supporting the role of advanced practice nurses, states that this study captures "both the promise of advanced practice nursing as well as the shortcoming of the present health care delivery system."

"Nursing is certainly recognized as one of the independent health professions" according to Kraus (1992) who writes about barriers to practice and reimbursement. However, advanced practice nurses providing community-based care recognize the importance of connecting with other health care providers and with acute care agencies. Consistent with this philosophy, the entrepreneurial CNC practices described in this chapter were developed by entering into contracts and developing joint ventures with agencies already providing services in the rural area. This chapter will focus on the evolution of an autonomous innovative rural practice that a nurse practitioner has developed through the University of Rochester Community Nursing Center (CNC) that is poised to address access, cost effectiveness, and quality care for underserved populations.

THE UNIVERSITY OF ROCHESTER COMMUNITY NURSING CENTER

Historically, a number of different faculty practice models have been used and continue to influence the development of academic nursing centers today. Potash and Taylor (1993) identify four examples: unification, collaboration, the integrated model, and the entrepreneurial model. Unification is usually described at the University of Rochester and Rush Presbyterian, where administration of clinical agencies and the school of nursing are "unified" and faculty practice as both clinicians and educators. A newer approach, the entrepreneurial model, encourages faculty members to design their own practices, which may also provide opportunities for teaching or research. Examples of this type of model are described at the University of Tennessee at Memphis (Potash & Taylor, 1993) and in the University of Rochester Community Nursing Center (Walker, 1994).

The University of Rochester CNC was subsequently developed as an entrepreneurial model within the context of "unification" as a broad, comprehensive model designed to foster a variety of self-supporting satellite faculty practices. This is consistent with the literature on intrepreneuring. According to Hollander, Allen, and Mechanic (1992) "the intrepreneur is the intracorporate entrepreneur." These authors also identify benefits to intrepreneuring in an established organization such as the University of Rochester School of Nursing, which include contributing to an organization's competitive edge and positively influencing recruitment and retention. It is a cost-effective way for implementing new program goals. The organization of the CNC as a professional corporation also facilitated opportunities for faculty and students to learn and integrate sound business practices into nursing practice. Figure 1 indicates important business functions that have become

Figure 1 Business functions.

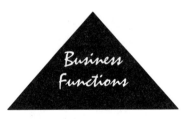

▲   Corporation Management

▲   Business Planning

▲   Project/Program Budgeting

▲   Marketing

▲   Entrepreneuring

▲   Financial Analysis

part of faculty development and content for student education at the University of Rochester School of Nursing.

The University of Rochester CNC, developed as a "center without walls" to provide opportunities for diverse and autonomous faculty practice in the community has already been described in Chapter 5. There were three important reasons for this futuristic approach of a "center without walls": (1) the University of Rochester faculty have a rich history with faculty practice and the populations served were very diverse; (2) community needs of underserved populations in the Rochester and surrounding areas were diverse—in both urban and rural areas; and (3) the philosophy of the CNC was to improve access to care by establishing nurse-managed practices in close proximity to home, work, or schools through partnerships and joint entrepreneurial ventures with community agencies. Development of diverse satellite faculty practices to provide access to care, particularly in rural communities is well supported in the nursing literature. Nurse practitioners, practicing in rural areas and with populations such as the elderly, inmates, and HIV-infected people increase client access to care. Additionally, the faculty practice described in this chapter consists of three practice sites and is an excellent example of the evolution of an entrepreneurial, autonomous self-supporting practice.

EVOLUTION OF THE RURAL PRACTICES WITHIN THE CNC

The struggles and successes of developing this autonomous, entrepreneurial practice for the nurse practitioner (NP) author are consistent with problems that nurse practitioners have historically had in trying to serve underserved populations. Barger and Rosenfeld (1993) write that at a time when it is difficult to attract enough primary care physicians to underserved rural and inner-city areas, nurse practitioners are experiencing significant barriers. This portion of the chapter will describe chronologically the development of three rural practices and the entrepreneurial satellite faculty practice developed through the University of Rochester School of Nursing CNC.

Attempts by the NP author to provide primary care actually began in 1985, when this NP moved his family to rural Wyoming County in western New York to take a position as a family nurse practitioner in a local community health care center (CCHCC). After two years, the position was eliminated when the practice was converted to a physician private practice. Subsequently, the NP secured a pediatric nurse practitioner position at another community health center (Oak Orchard Community Health Center) near Brockport, New York, approximately forty-five miles from home. He worked in this setting for slightly more than four years. During that time, individuals and families would come to the practitioner's home, seeking health care. The patients had to be turned away since there were no official linkages with a medical back-up as required by New York state law. "The decision to open a nurse practitioner practice is often difficult to make. Success depends on the possession of specific resources, such as adequate skills, finances, emotional support, and the desire to be one's own boss," according to Calmelat (1993). Although the NP was interested in developing his own practice, certain barriers prevented this from happening at that time.

After about two years at the community health center in Brockport, the medical director of the center agreed to consult with the NP to provide the required support of the practice for those patients seen after hours in rural Wyoming County. However, this arrangement was not very satisfactory. There were problems with the distance between locations of the practice sites and the paperwork necessary to alter the certificate of need used by the health center to incorporate the rural practice in Wyoming County. The elusive goal of establishing a private practice and providing primary care in the rural area was again meeting with barriers and discouragement.

In late 1990, the nurse practitioner contacted the Associate Dean and Director of Community Centered Practice (second author) in the newly established University of Rochester CNC. Here the potential for development of an autonomous rural practice was perceived as a possibility and a goal under the umbrella of the CNC. There was a desire to demonstrate new and innovative roles for advance nursing practice in the community and an interest in bringing more nurse practitioners on as clinical faculty. However, since there was no immediate opportunity for financial support and connection to physicians in the rural community, this was established as a goal for the future—to be pursued as soon as financially feasible.

During that time, the Senior Health Service, a nurse-managed clinic designed to serve the well elderly in downtown Rochester had opened through a joint effort with the Regional Council on Aging. This practice needed a nurse practitioner with experience and became an ideal bridging practice to support the NP until the dream of a rural practice could be developed. The NP agreed to help develop this urban entrepreneurial, autonomous practice and use the opportunity to sharpen entrepreneurial skills, business expertise, and to develop the first satellite faculty practice under the CNC.

"There are at least five different ways to finance a nursing center: contracts, fee for service, third-party reimbursement, charities, and grants," according to Elsberry and Nelson (1993, p. 408). Salary support for this SHS practice, initially was primarily supported through a private grant. However, the grant facilitated the bridging between this practice and hopefully a more viable, longer term financially supported practice to be developed in the rural community.

During the 1991 academic year, in the rural community, the NP explored future opportunities to develop some type of financially supported, autonomous satellite faculty practice under the CNC. An opportunity presented itself through the Wyoming County Health Department. Although this was not the original plan for an office-based primary care practice, it provided the opportunity to establish the NP as a recognized practitioner in the health care community in Wyoming County.

PRACTICE IN COUNTY JAIL

The director of the Wyoming County Health Department had chosen to hire a NP on a part-time basis to replace the physician who had formerly provided care to the inmates in the county jail. The NP had established a relationship with this individual previously in the community and she was interested in a nurse practitioner model of care for the following reasons:

1. She was interested in providing health care and health promotion services to the inmates;
2. The county was interested in reducing the cost of providing care in the county budget; and
3. She was aware that the NP was interested in developing autonomous practice roles in the rural community.

The director's and the NP's objectives were accomplished through the development of this nurse-managed practice in a number of ways. Since the county needed only part-time assistance, the CNC affiliation allowed this to become the first step in building an entrepreneurial faculty practice and the nurse practitioner could establish a more holistic practice with the inmates.

The county jail was a two-year-old facility that had the capacity to hold 60 inmates. This represented more beds than were projected for the community's needs. Consequently, the excess beds were built into the facility to provide additional income to the county. The "extra beds" were and continue to be used to house federal inmates awaiting trial or for temporary housing prior to their incarceration in a federal facility. The jail currently maintains a census of approximately 4 to 45 inmates. The facility houses both male and female inmates, and the number of inmates seen per session has varied from 5 to 18. The CNC faculty practice contract specifies no more than two sessions per week be dedicated to this practice.

The previous physician who provided care in the jail had no charting system, kept insufficient records, and billed the county a fee per individual inmate seen. The NP has subsequently developed a documentation system that was available on site during the period of inmate incarceration. The documentation system provides a holistic approach to care, with attention to the physiological, psychosocial, and emotional needs of the inmates. NP interventions, health education, and referrals for care by other providers, and recording of ongoing treatment is now a part of the documentation system. This chart is also pulled in case a released inmate should return. The goal of health education was met by both the NP and the county community health nurses. Currently, county health nurses come into the jail to do tuberculosis programs and AIDS testing. Other health education is done on an individual basis by the NP.

The goal of reducing costs has also been achieved in a number of ways. The contract through the CNC is designed on an hourly rate, rather than by number of inmates seen. Also, the use of controlled drugs and the utilization of diagnostic testing of inmates out of the facility has dramatically been reduced. Another benefit to the inmates and to the county is the development of collaborative communications between the NP, the mental health counselor, and the psychiatrist. There is now a more deliberate and consistent approach to mental health issues.

The following patient-care situations provide an example of improved collaboration and care provided in the county jail. This case discussion also reflects how practitioners in the rural community can provide holistic, family-centered care because of the opportunity to provide care to more than one family member in more than one setting. Although this case history is intended to reflect outcomes related to care of inmates in the county jail, the description of care provided to the inmate's mother in another rural practice (same locale) contribute to the richness and rewards of rural health care.

JM was a 22-year-old white male, who was followed over time in the infirmary at the Wyoming County Jail. The first few times JM was seen by the NP for upper respiratory symptoms.

After getting more comfortable with the practitioner, he began to talk about periods when he would "blank out." He said that people would be talking to him, but he would not hear them. He also stated that when he had been arrested, he did not remember his activities and felt that he needed to agree with what the police were saying.

The NP had previously provided care to his mother (see below) at one of the other NP offices, and she had voiced some concerns about JM. She reported that an uncle of JM had similar symptoms and was diagnosed with seizures and had responded well to medications. A neurological evaluation was arranged for JM and all testing was normal. At this time, the psychiatric counsellor and the NP met to discuss JM and develop a treatment plan. The NP continued to provide care periodically in the infirmary, and JM began regular visits with the counsellor. After about one month of therapy, JM was able to discuss the fact that he had been abused by an uncle and a foster father. His symptoms were improved and since his release he has been able to maintain a job. Also, he will be married soon.

JM's mother PJ is a 40-year-old caucasian female who first started to come to the NP for recurrent sinus infections. Since she was married to a farmer and the family was self-employed, it was not only difficult for PJ to make appointments during the day, but also difficult to meet family expenses based on their limited income. After several visits in a short period of time, PJ was referred to an allergist for skin testing and probable hyposensitization shots. The allergist concurred with the evaluation and the allergy shots were started.

Since PJ was seen for primary care in the off hours, there was opportunity to spend time with her during the waiting period after her allergy shots. During this time, and in subsequent visits, PJ began to provide more information regarding the family history. This information included not only a history of being abused as a young child and adolescent, but also the fact that both of her children had been abused. Both abuses were reported to be by family members as well as a foster parent with whom the children had been placed for a short period of time.

She also provided information regarding events leading up to JM's arrest and his episodes of incarceration. During these conversations, she discussed the fact that JM did not remember any information about the acts that lead him to be arrested. She went on to explain about the uncle who had similar episodes. Based on this information, the NP initiated a neurologic evaluation and case conferenced this patient with the social worker at the county jail in order to obtain counseling for JM.

During these allergy shot visits, PJ also discussed that her daughter was dating a man who had been incarcerated for sexual abuse. During this time, PJ received counseling and health education by the NP on how to approach her daughter regarding this issue. Subsequently, PJ has become more empowered as a parent and is involved with a group of mothers who have taken a vocal role in the community to encourage judges to sentence molesters to stiffer penalties.

FAMILY HEALTH CARE PRACTICE

The second satellite faculty practice that was developed in the rural area was established through a joint venture with the Wyoming County Community Hospital (WCCH). The Family Health Care Center, a practice site owned by the hospital, had no primary care provider. The center office was located in Attica, New York, a rural village in northwest Wyoming County and southeast Genessee County. It had been difficult to recruit physicians to that area; and one area physician had retired. Attica was clearly an underserved area, and compounding the problem, had a growing population. After negotiating a contract with the hospital which stipulated that the hospital would provide and maintain the space, provide medical back-up according to state law, pay an appropriate salary, and include a productivity bonus consistent with physician contracts, the NP practice began in that site in July 1992. Initially, the practitioner was hired on a part-time basis, with incremental increases in time and financial support built into the contract as the patient population increased. Shortly thereafter, an internist was hired for that site full time. He practiced there for six months (as a totally separate practice) and then left for an urban setting.

After the first physician left, another internist was hired. Both he and the NP have continued to practice in that site in separate practices. The physician at that site is not the medical back-up for the practitioner since the NP requires consulting physicians to support a family nurse practitioner role. During this time, the NP practice has continued to grow to the point of approximately 200 patient visits a month with five one-half day clinical sessions per week. The practice is a family practice with a wide range of patients including several home-bound patients who require house calls. However, family care and care of children are also an important part of this practice. An example of the primary care provided and collaboration with other providers is described next.

SB is an 18-month-old female who has been followed by the NP since she was three weeks old. At that time, she presented with febrile illness. Upon examination, she was found to have bilateral otitis media and was treated with Amoxil. The infection cleared as documented by return examination. SB had a subsequent febrile illness in January 1993 and was diagnosed with a urinary tract infection. This was also resolved with Amoxil. However, due to her age and the extent of her symptoms, SB was referred to a pediatric urologist and found to have gradual vesicoureteral reflux on the left. She has been subsequently managed in the NP practice based upon recommendations made by the urologist. She has had no further episodes since that time.

At her well-child visit at seven months of age, SB demonstrated an exotropia and was referred to the ophthalmologist. Treatment was recommended, however, her parents have refused patching despite many discussions about it. At her last visit, SB was developmentally delayed and her weight curve has dropped from 95 percent to 25 percent. She is now waiting further evaluation at the tertiary pediatric center close to the rural area. This description describes the need for and use of physician colleagues when appropriate.

RURAL MOBILE HEALTH UNIT

The last rural practice that became part of this entrepreneurial faculty practice began as an extension of the Wyoming County Community Hospital contract. During the negotiations for the Attica primary health care clinic, the NP and hospital CEO discussed the NP's ideas for expanding the NP role into other practices. The hospital organization had a 38-foot recreational vehicle, used to transport executives to and from conferences. Initially, the hospital wanted to sell this van. The NP and CEO discussed the possibility of converting this vehicle into an office on wheels. Thus, the Wyoming County Mobile Health Unit was born. In the spring of 1993, the council members met to investigate the feasibility of locating the mobile health van in particular areas.

In July, the council members of a local township were contacted to investigate the feasibility of locating the mobile health unit in their area. Also, in July, the mobile health unit set up next to a town recreation building in one of the surrounding villages which happened to be the site of an old public school. However, despite advertisements and presentations at public meetings, the utilization of the mobile health unit was low. In the fall, concern turned to what would be done in the snowy months ahead and the local volunteer fire department was contacted and arrangements were made to locate the unit in front of the fire house. This move provided the mobile unit with several advantages. First, it provided a site that was more visible to the public and has subsequently increased the daily census. The second advantage was that it provided the NP and the mobile van with a form of communication with the community. At the original site there was no conventional phone hook-up and the van was located in a "no service" area for the mobile phone. Over the past seven months, the daily census has grown from two or three patients to eleven per day with patients now receiving their primary care through the unit. Although the individual practices still fit well under the cluster of service "longer term continuity of care," with the three entrepreneurial practices making up on financially supported faculty practice, this care now more clearly fits under Services to Organizations, Businesses, and Health Care Providers.

CONCLUSIONS

"The first challenge is to think and act with the perseverance and determination of an entrepreneur" Walker (1994). This chapter represents the entrepreneurial spirit of both the NP author and the CNC organization and the use of entrepreneurial and intrepreneurial skills to finally achieve the goal of a financially supported, autonomous, rural primary care practice. According to Vogel and Doleysh (1988), entrepreneurs take only moderate risks and consistently use skill, judgment, resources, and data to make decisions with predictable outcomes. As a clinical faculty member in the University of Rochester CNC, this NP author also contributes to the educational mission by teaching periodic classes to masters students and had consistently precepted a student in the nurse practitioner graduate program.

The University of Rochester School of Nursing's CNC continues to explore creative and innovative ways to make a practice like the one described in this chapter a reality for interested practitioners. Contracts such as this one are negotiated between organizations in the community (such as the Wyoming County Hospital and the Wyoming County Health Department) and the CNC for nurse practitioner and other professional nursing services (see Figure 2). According to the terms of the contract, the community agencies pay the CNC for the practitioner services, so the practitioner is a clinical faculty member of the CNC. Contracts such as this one allow for the development of diverse practices as described in this chapter, while

Figure 2   Organizations, businesses and health care providers.

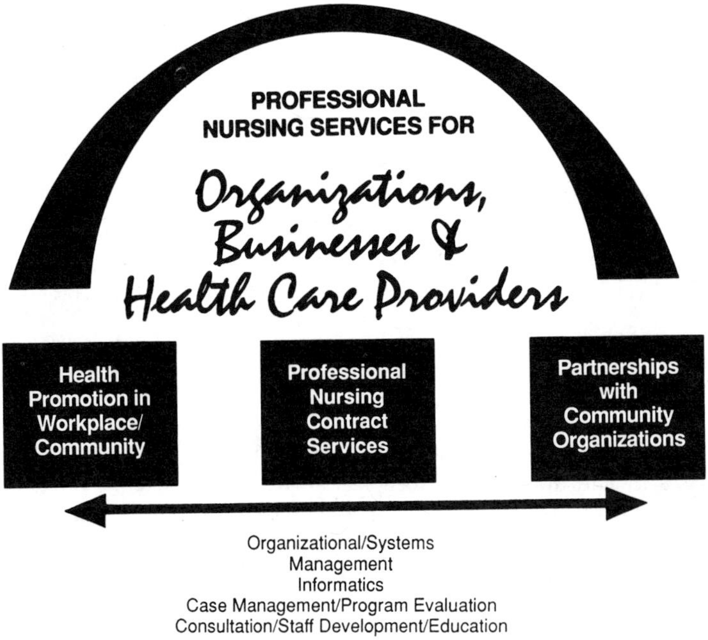

All rights reserved

generating sufficient revenue to support the faculty practice role of the faculty member. This contract payment structure and bridging from one practice to another has proven to be financially successful for both the CNC as an organization and for the individual faculty member. The University of Rochester CNC administrator's reasons for choosing contract payment for faculty practice are consistent with those cited by Elsberry and Nelson (1993). These reasons include: (1) contracts provide opportunities for reasonable planning for the future of the practitioner and the CNC; (2) fees and services can be preestablished, consequently the practitioner and the CNC can negotiate a consistent, predictable salary; and (3) the scope of the services needed by an organization can more effectively be matched with a particular faculty practitioner's expertise.

The development of this entrepreneurial satellite faculty practice has been a significant challenge. Roadblocks and barriers consistently thwarted an individual nurse practitioner's and the CNC administrator's efforts to establish a rural practice. Barger and Rosenfeld (1993) state the problem well, "One can only conclude that nurses want to practice in these settings. And yet, our existing health policy decrees that somehow the public will be better served and quality of care will be improved if reimbursement and prescriptive authority flow through another provider who does not even choose to be in that setting."

REFERENCES

Avorn, J., Everitt, D., & Baker, M. (1991). The neglected medical history and therapeutic choices for abdominal pain: A nationwide study of 799 physicians and nurses. *Archives of Internal Medicine, 151*, 694.

Barger, S., & Rosenfeld, P. (1993). Models in community health care: Findings from a national study of community nursing centers. *Nursing and Health Care, 14*(8), 426–431.

Bessman, A. (1974). Comparison of medical care in nurse clinician and physician clinics in medical school affiliated hospitals. *Journal of Chronic Disease, 27*, 15–125.

Brown, S., & Grimes, D. (1993). Nurse Practitioners and Certified Nurse Midwives. *A meta-analysis of studies on nurses in primary care roles.* Washington, DC: American Nurses Publishing.

Calmelat, A. (1993). Tips for starting your own nurse practitioner practice. *Nurse Practitioner, 18*(4), 58.

Campbell, J., Mauksch, H., Heikirk, H., & Hosokawa, M. (1990). Collaborative practice and provider styles of delivering health care. *Social Science Medicine, 30*, 1359–1365.

Chambers, L., & West, A. (1978). The St. John's randomized trial of the family practice nurse: Health outcomes of patients. *International Journal of Epidemiology, 7*, 153–161.

Charney, E., & Kitzman, H. (1971). The child health nurse (Pediatric Nurse Practitioner) in private practice: A controlled trial. *New England Journal of Medicine, 285*, 1353–1358.

Chen, S., Barkauskas, V., Ohlson, V., Chen, E., & DeStefano, L. (1983). Health problems encountered by pediatric nurse practitioners and pediatricians in ambulatory care clinics. *Medical Care, 21,* 168–179.

Elsberry, N., & Nelson, F. (1993). How to plan financial support for nursing centers. *Nursing and Health Care, 14*(8), 408–414.

Goodman, H., & Perrin, E. (1978). Evening telephone management by nurse practitioners and physicians. *Nursing Research, 27,* 233–237.

Hollander, S. F., Allen, K. D., & Mechanic, J. (1992). The intrapreneurial nursing department: Nature and nurture. *Nursing Economics, 10,* 1.

Komaroff, A., Sawayer, K., Flatley, M., & Browne, C. (1976). Nurse practitioner management of common respiratory and genitourinary infections, using protocols. *Nursing Research, 25*(2), 84–89.

Kraus, J. (1992). Regulation of advanced practice nursing—The cog in the health policy engine. *Journal of Professional Nursing, 8*(4), 200.

Lewis, C., & Resnick, B. (1967). Nurse clinics and progressive ambulatory patient care. *The New England Journal of Medicine, 277,* 236–241.

Lewis, C., Resnick, B., Schmidt, G., & Waxman, L. (1969). Activities, events and outcomes in ambulatory patient care. *The New England Journal of Medicine, 280,* 645–649.

McLaughlin, F., Anderson, S., Cesa, T., Larson, P., Johnson, H., Gibson, J., Lemons, M., & Delucchi, K. (1979). Nurse practitioners', public health nurses', and physician performance of clinical simulation test: COPD. *Western Journal of Nursing Research, 1,* 275–295.

McLaughlin, F., Cesa, T., Johnson, H., Lemons, M., Anderson, S., Larson, P., & Gibson, J. (1979). Nurses' and physicians' performance on clinical simulation test: Hypertension. *Research in Nursing and Health, 2,* 61–72.

Perrin, E., & Goodman, H. (1978). Telephone management of acute pediatric illnesses. *The New England Journal of Medicine, 298,* 130–135.

Potash, M., & Taylor, D. (1993). *Nursing faculty practice: Models and methods.* National Organization of Nurse Practitioner Faculties. Pp. 6–7.

Ramsay, J., McKenzie, J., & Fish, D. (1982). Physicians and nurse practitioners: Do they provide equivalent health care? *American Journal of Public Health, 72,* 55–57.

Safriet, B. (1992). Health care dollars and regulatory sense: The role of advanced practice nursing. *The Yale Journal on Regulation, 9*, 417–488.

Scherer, K., Fortin, F., Spitzer, W., & Kergin, D. (1977). Nurse practitioner in primary care. VII. A cohort study of 99 nurses and 79 associated physicians. *Canadian Medical Association Journal, 116*, 856–862.

Spitzer, W., Sackett, D., Sibley, J., Roberts, R., Gent, M., Kergin, D., Hackett, D., & Olynich, A. (1974). The Burlington Randomized Trial of the nurse practitioner. *The New England Journal of Medicine, 290*, 251–256.

Stein, G. (1972). The Use of nurse practitioner in the management of patients with diabetes mellitus. *Medical Care, 12*, 885–890.

Vogel, G., & Doleysh, N. (1988) *Entrepreneuring: A nurse's guide to starting a business* (p. 27). New York: National League for Nursing Press.

Walker, P. H. (1994). A comprehensive community nursing center model: Maximizing practice income—A challenge to educators. *Journal of Professional Nursing, 10*(3), 133–139.

9

Opportunities and Obstacles: Development of a True Collaborative Practice with Physicians

Colleen M. Dwyer
Patricia Hinton Walker
Anthony Suchman
Peter Coggiola

The best model—one that reduces costs while enhancing quality and comprehensiveness—is collaborative practice.

Mundinger, 1994

*T*he National Joint Practice Commission of 1972 defined joint practice as "nurses and physicians collaborating as colleagues to provide patient care." With the advent of health care reform, the topic of partnerships and collaborative practice between nurse practitioners and physicians becomes even more important. According to Mundinger, (1994, p. 211) "collaborative practice is more comprehensive, most cost effective, and therefore more competitive than independent practice." Mundinger (1994, p. 213) further states that "the best model—one that reduces costs while enhancing quality and comprehensiveness— is collaborative practice." The focus of the chapter will be on the process of development of a true collaborative practice rather than a traditional setting where the nurse practitioner "works for" the physician. This chapter will describe a collaborative practice that was developed as part of a community nursing center faculty practice at the University of Rochester School of Nursing.

Community Nursing Centers (CNCs) are still considered a new and innovative delivery model that provides consumers direct access to professional nursing services. These services usually include primary care, prevention, and health promotion services. Nurse-managed care is a term frequently used to describe the practices in nursing centers, however, it is in this context and through a nursing center that this collaborative practice developed. In this case, the result is effective comanagement of care of patients at a hospital-based primary care practice at Highland Hospital in Rochester, New York, and at a nurse-managed site (the Senior Health Service) that is part of the University of Rochester CNC.

THE UNIVERSITY OF ROCHESTER CNC

The University of Rochester School of Nursing has a long history of integrating education and practice through the unification model. Early linkages for clinical faculty were primarily in Strong Memorial Hospital, where many practitioners could be described in some ways as participating on a daily basis in some form of collaboration with faculty members and students from the school of medicine. However, with the development of the Community Nursing Center, there have been increasing opportunities for more autonomous faculty practice outside the medical center and the hospital. Moccia (1993) encourages "a faculty of the community" where loyalty shifts from traditional hospital nursing to alliances with the community. The practice described in this chapter is a form of a new type of alliance with a community and reflects a model for truly collaborative practice relationships between nurse practitioners and physician groups.

The University of Rochester CNC was organized as a faculty group practice and its comprehensive services have already been described in Chapter 5. The faculty practice described in this chapter evolved out of a nurse-managed practice for the elderly called the Senior Health Service. This nurse practitioner managed practice was the first practice developed under the CNC service cluster, Services for Longer Term Continuity of Care, (see Figure 1).

Figure 1 Longer term continuity of care.

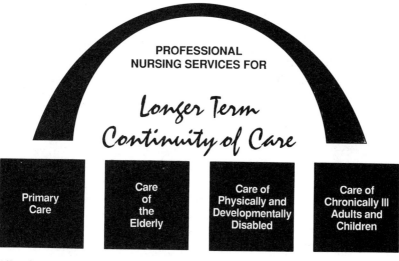

PROFESSIONAL
NURSING SERVICES FOR

*Longer Term
Continuity of Care*

| Primary Care | Care of the Elderly | Care of Physically and Developmentally Disabled | Care of Chronically Ill Adults and Children |

DEVELOPMENT OF THE TRUE
COLLABORATIVE PRACTICE

The Senior Health Service (SHS) opened in the fall of 1991. A nurse practitioner, Peter Coggolia, with a number of years of experience, began to establish an autonomous practice on the sixth floor of the Regional Council on Aging building. Initially, neither the nurse practitioner (NP), nor the physician had experience with autonomous nurse practitioner practice. Consequently, during the early days, the NP established a format for consultation meetings with the consulting MD. Prior to that time, the meetings had a teacher-student approach. Efforts were made for the NP to develop case studies based on a specific patient or patients, provide background information, and present potential plans of care. Then, at the meetings with the consulting MD, the NP would present options and discuss the benefits/drawbacks of each joint plan of care. Through this approach, guidelines were established for when and if consultation was needed for clinical decision making.

Even though the SHS was located within the main building for the Regional Council on Aging (RCOA), many of the seniors who attended the agency offerings were not aware the nurse-managed practice existed. A second approach was needed to increase the visibility of the SHS within the target client population. To accomplish this, a series of educational programs were presented at the nutrition center, housed on the first floor of the RCOA building. These educational programs were eventually expanded to several of the high-rise apartments in the downtown area where senior citizens lived. During that same timeframe, the public health nurse who was assigned to the RCOA building was required to cut back her overall practice time. With the change, the monthly blood pressure checks that she had performed were incorporated into the SHS practice.

In the fall of 1992, the SHS practitioner offered to participate in the medicare demonstration project that was studying the promotion of immunizing seniors for influenza. The SHS took this program to the majority of the senior high-rises in the city as well as a few in the suburbs surrounding Rochester. Utilizing this program, the SHS staff was able to provide immunizations sessions for 350 to 450 seniors per year, while marketing the services of the CNC.

There were also opportunities to interface with other agencies who had frustrations about helping seniors they worked with get health care or health assessments. These agencies started referring seniors who were home bound for various reasons to SHS for house calls. Many of these visits were for patients living in federally mandated health manpower shortage areas.

As the practice began to take shape, it became a priority to work with physicians who could accept and understand the more autonomous role of the NP. Working with the original physician associated with the practice, the NP took on more responsibility for case management as well as primary care. The outcome was that the meetings became more streamlined and more patient focused. The end result was a more comfortable relationship with the physician. Consequently, the NP was able to take a more central role in the development and delivery of patient care.

After about six months, it became necessary to recruit a new physician as a consultant, since the first physician decided to start attending a PhD program. The new consultant was selected using an interview process. This new consulting arrangement was with a group of three physicians. Initially, meetings were set up with the NP and all three physicians. However, this format became difficult due to conflicting schedules. There were many details to be worked out with three physicians. One area of concern was which service SHS patients would be admitted to when patients required hospitalization. After discussion with the group, it was decided that the MD consultants would rotate on a one- to three-month basis, depending on call schedules and teaching responsibilities.

The changes in physician consultant required that trust in clinical judgment be rebuilt. This was accomplished in much the same way as it had been developed with the original consultant. As the relationship developed further, less time was needed and meetings were less frequent. Face-to-face discussions were supplemented with telephone conversations and consultations as needed.

In the summer of 1993, the initiating NP had an opportunity to develop a rural entrepreneurial practice. Another practitioner, Colleen Dwyer, was recruited into the practice. At the same time, the primary physician consultant expressed interest in the development of a true collaborative practice. In this new practice, the NP would continue the SHS practice on a part-time basis, and the rest of her practice would be a new collaborative practice role within the physician group practice at Highland Hospital.

Development of the New Collaborative Practice

This new innovative role between Highland Hospital and the Senior Health Service became a reality in the fall of 1993. After several meetings between the new NP, the physician group, and the CNC administrator, the preliminary details of this role were developed. The NP clinical faculty member's time would be split between the SHS and the practice at Highland Hospital. The primary advantage of this joint venture was the flexibility for role development. The mutually set goals for this position were to: (1) further develop a collaborative practice model utilizing the adult nurse practitioner; (2) initiate a patient education program that would benefit patients at both practices; (3) become involved in teaching residents and ancillary staff about the role of the NP; and (4) further enhance the role of the NP in the provision of primary, secondary, and tertiary prevention according to the Neuman Systems Model (Neuman, 1982).

One of the early objectives in the development of this collaborative practice was to develop mutual respect for the different abilities, knowledge, and skills that each respective discipline would bring to the practice. The building of trust would be required to make this new "collaborative practice" role a success. The focus of care provided by the NP would be nursing-centered.

NURSE PRACTITIONER AND PHYSICIAN EXPECTATIONS

Nurse Practitioner Expectations

The application of holistic care is a critical focus of the nurse practitioner's education at the master's level and NPs are prepared to provide care that encompasses the entire family unit. Holistic care is crucial in today's health care system. Health professionals must refocus energy not on acute care but on prevention. The Neuman Systems Model provides a basis for the focus on prevention. Neuman emphasized that the client and family are the center of the application of holistic care. The whole person is addressed utilizing five variables for assessment: spiritual, sociocultural, developmental, physiological, and psychoemotional. Within the Neuman model, it is the provider's responsibility to assist the patient to develop lines of resistance and lines of defense to prevent breakdown of any or all of the variables. (See Figure 2.) Examples of primary prevention include health maintenance, health promotion, and education. Case management of selected clients who were home bound was also a key element in this NP practice.

The responsibility of tertiary prevention also lies within the scope of the NP. The Senior Health Service serves a population of patients that benefit from tertiary prevention services as described by Neuman. Patients seen at this site not only have multiple medical diagnoses, but also have limited access to health care resources. The NP is crucial in the coordination of health care for these patients. Services provided at this site include the provision of both primary and tertiary prevention ranging from routine health maintenance to acute care visits. Case studies presented later in this chapter will describe the

Figure 2 Neuman interdisciplinary practice.

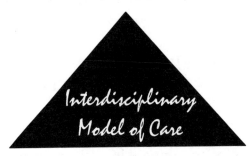

NEUMAN HEALTH SYSTEMS MODEL

▲ Mutual Goal Setting Between Client and Provider
▲ Focus of Care Consistent with Community Based Practice
 Primary and Tertiary Prevention as Intervention
▲ Holistic Approach with Attention to:

Stressors	Variables	
Intrapersonal	Physiological	Psychological
Interpersonal	Developmental	Spiritual
Extrapersonal	Sociocultural	

application of the Neuman Systems Model to patient care in this collaborative practice.

Physician Expectations

From the physician perspective, a number of key elements were required for success of the collaborative role. First, all participants (nurse practitioners and physicians alike) must be committed to shake off the more traditional assumptions about doctor-nurse relationships. Second, all participants would need to believe that teams do better than individuals and provide better care than one discipline can do alone. Additionally, the position must be constructed in such as way as to demonstrate partnership and parody. Thus lines of supervision are similar for physicians and for the nurse practitioners within the unit. Faculty ranks for both the nurse practitioner (as a clinical faculty member in the School of Nursing) should be comparable with the physician faculty members who are faculty members in the School of Medicine. Consequently, participation (by the nurse practitioner clinical faculty member) in teaching, administrative activities of the unit, and in Highland Hospital medical faculty meetings would not only be invited, but expected. A third element is that the nurse practitioners have their own panels (or groups) of patients for whom they are the primary care providers, just as the physicians have their own panel. Last, practitioners of both disciplines should help each other through consultation in areas pertaining to each discipline's specific professional expertise. Also, in general, both medical and nurse practitioner faculty would assist with cross-coverage during periods of absence.

Additional expectations of the role from the physician included: (1) providing quality primary care; (2) working independently within the scope of one's area of competence—asking for assistance when care moves outside of that zone; (3) offering assistance to physicians with areas that are outside their area of competence; (4) having the self-confidence to make unsolicited suggestions in the spirit of partnership and teamwork; and (5) seeking to become involved in all of the unit's activities and willingness to participate in the long-term planning of the unit.

Guidelines for Practice and Education

The guidelines established for this practice were within this context of a holistic, nursing-centered approach to care. It was agreed that the NP expectations would function as outlined in the American Academy of Nurse Practitioner's "Scope of Practice," and a collaborative practice agreement was established with the collaborating physician accordingly. The following guidelines were developed with assistance/approval of those who would play an integral part in the future and success of this new practice. These guidelines were an actual part of the collaborative agreement and were available to all those who worked in the clinic:

1. The NP/MD would work collaboratively in the provision of care of patients seen at Highland Hospital and the Senior Health Service.
2. The NP would have emergent access to the physician for medical back-up while at the SHS.
3. The NP would orient the current staff (practice manager, nursing staff, and secretaries) to the role of the NP in primary care.
4. The NP would act as a liaison for the development of the role within the Highland Department of Medicine and the residency clinic.
5. The NP would have a faculty appointment within the residency program and conduct educational sessions for the residents.
6. The NP would develop a comprehensive educational program to promote health maintenance and wellness for patients in the practice and the community.

Another step in the development of this collaborative practice was the education of not only the residents, but the ancillary staff to the role of the NP. This would be achieved through discussion with the office staff and the practice manager. Guidelines were established to outline which patients would be appropriate for the NP to see, and those that would require referral to the MD. Written information would also be developed and was provided to reinforce this guideline. Information would then be disseminated to patients when the NP would be responsible for their first visit and this would be done prior to the patient visit.

OPPORTUNITIES AND OBSTACLES

Opportunities

This multifaceted role brings with it many opportunities. The key questions that need to be identified include whether the opportunities as supported by the literature and the projected health care reform objectives are relevant to this practice. This collaborative practice and the opportunity to provide care along the health illness continuum (see Figure 3), would be one of the highlights of this practice. Also, this role has the opportunity to bring the adult nurse practitioner role into the forefront of health care reform.

Cost-effectiveness is one issue that arises when looking at new opportunities for the adult nurse practitioners. Will this practice meet the challenge? Mundinger (1994, p. 212) emphasizes that "teams of primary care physicians and nurse practitioners are even more cost effective and comprehensive." A number of other authors have reviewed the issue of cost-effective care provided by nurse practitioners. A meta-analysis by Brown and Grimes (1993) confirms the effectiveness of the NP in primary health care. Multiple studies have demonstrated the effectiveness of the NP in the primary care arena (Bessman, 1974; Brown & Grimes, 1993; Charney & Kitzman, 1971; Lewis

Figure 3 Continuum of care.

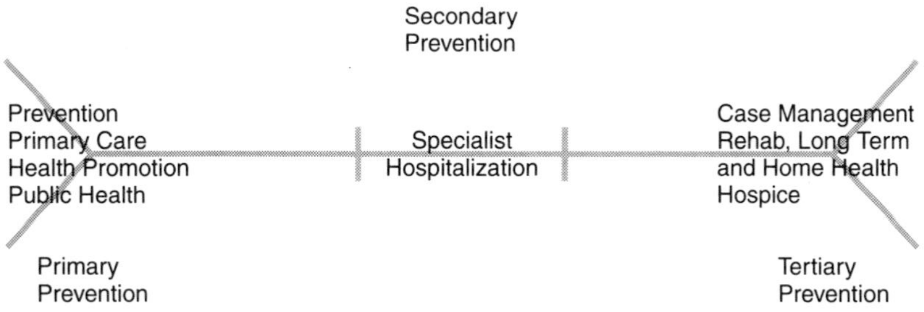

Neuman Systems Model

& Resnick, 1967; and McLaughlin et al., 1979). Avorn, Everitt, and Baker, (1991) indicated that the NP was more likely than MDs to incorporate issues such as diet, psychosocial, and cost concerns into the care. These components are key elements in the objective of current health care reform.

Cost-effectiveness of a practice can also be supported through appropriate management of primary, secondary, and tertiary prevention as described by Neuman (1982). To meet the challenge of health care reform in the context of managed care, effective interventions in the primary and tertiary prevention categories can achieve a cost savings by reducing the more expensive costs of acute care, usually associated with secondary prevention (see Figure 4). Appropriateness of care, much of it enhanced by collaborative practice, can reduce costs and decrease dollars spent on acute care visits.

From the physician's perspective, the role would be conceptualized as an opportunity to develop something between the free-standing independent nurse practitioner and the more traditional "physician-assistant" type of role. In this new model, the nurse practitioner and primary care physicians would work together as colleagues, providing primary care and preventive services as a team. The role was further conceptualized as an

Figure 4 Cost effectiveness.

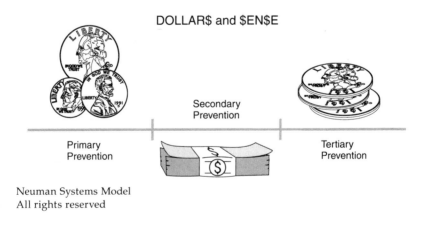

DOLLAR$ and ENE

Secondary
Prevention

Primary
Prevention

Tertiary
Prevention

Neuman Systems Model

important educational opportunity. This would provide medical residents with some experience of collaborative care and, at some point in the future, a similar learning opportunity for nurse practitioner students.

Obstacles

Through the phases of development and structure of this role, several "obstacles" became apparent. The expectations of the role were outlined previously, but there were still areas of adjustment. The presence of a nurse practitioner for the hospital-based clinic was not only new to some of the physicians, but to the staff as well. Education related to the role was interjected at all staff meetings, along with written information provided on a monthly basis to reinforce this new role. However, there was still some lack of understanding of the role.

Highland Hospital had six physicians that saw patients on the East 5 clinic, where this new role was to be implemented. Approximately 20 medical residents also see patients in this clinic. The main obstacle was role definition to this group of residents who were a culturally diverse group. None of the residents had worked with a NP in the past and confusion regarding the role was apparent at the first meeting. Utilizing individual sessions and written information regarding the role and responsibilities of the NP provided by the American Academy of Nurse Practitioners was beneficial.

With one exception, the six physicians that worked in the clinic (mentioned earlier) also had limited experience with an NP. The fact that this NP author had eight years of acute care clinical experience was a distinct advantage in gaining their trust and confidence. Over time and with much coaxing, acute care patients that were in these physician's practices were seen by the NP in the clinic. The biggest problem was the amount of time it took to obtain trust in clinical judgment.

Another obstacle was the chronicity of the patients referred from the SHS. A concern that was raised during the developmental phase of the role was the chronic patient population at the SHS. These patients were traditionally referred to the SHS practice either through Adult Protective or the Senior Center at the RCOA. Access to health care was extremely limited and in most cases absent. There was also concern about the time needed for patients from the SHS in order to make the site successful.

The first step in controlling the time involved from the physicians was to update the current files on the patients. This was done at the SHS and at Highland Hospital. A main objective was the streamlining of paper work and the continuity of charts between sites. Utilizing existing documentation forms from Highland allowed for continuity of clinical information. A database of charts was also established and updated at the hospital in case an acute care visit should require access to the information by the physician on call.

From the physician's perspective, the major obstacles are administrative and financial. There is not yet recognition of nurse practitioners as primary care providers by some HMOs and other payors. Current New York state regulations require medical affiliation in a manner that could be interpreted as the NP is subordinate. This problem continues to be further exacerbated by more flagrant regulations within some of the local HMOs in the Rochester area. These external constraints interfere with the external perception of partnership which, in turn, can perpetuate internal views and conflicts as well.

A second obstacle mentioned by the physician was financial. The question of how nurse practitioners are compensated when they do work that is similar to primary care physician's work remains quite controversial. There is a strong case for "equal pay for equal work," however this is a potential for problem for some physicians. By virtue of differences in education and training, primary care provided by physicians is likely to be somewhat different than that of nurse practitioners. These issues will require more honest and respectful dialogue to resolve.

A third obstacle related to the specific situation in which this collaborative practice was situated. It was difficult for one nurse practitioner to work with six attendings and 18 residents, providing all with an experience of collaborative team care. As opportunities present themselves in the future, the physician group clearly see the need to increase the number of nurse practitioners to take full advantage of the opportunity to learn more about true collaboration.

CARING, CURING, AND CASE STUDIES

Clients served by the Senior Health Service are an excellent example of a population with limited access and scarce health care dollars. The provision of health care to this population can be accomplished through a paradigm shift from curing to caring (Walker, 1993). This shift in paradigm would not only allow for the allocation of health care resources, but also focus on "caring" for these patients versus the "curing" mode that has become all too prevalent.

The application of the Neuman Systems Model has proven to be helpful to NPs and MDs as a way to focus on holistic family-centered care. The application of this model can best be represented through the use of a case study.

Case Study I: E.L. is a seventy-eight-year-old female patient with a past medical history of congestive heart failure, seizures, emphysema, s/p stroke, and dementia. Initial assessment of the patient occurred 5-91. Follow-up at this time was for routine health maintenance and tertiary prevention care. She was enrolled in an adult day-care program, and also has access to an emergency call system.

In 3-93, it became evident through several emergent office visits that E.L. was a subject of abuse from her family. At this point, adult protective services were utilized to monitor the situation. The client was competent to make her own decisions and elected to remain in the home. Support was given not only to the client, but also to those family members not involved with the abuse. Living with her granddaughter and grandson proved to be an ongoing struggle in order to provide care. The location of her home was also a concern not only from adult protective services, but also for the health care providers.

On 11-1-93, E.L. presented with an acute onset of respiratory distress which resulted in her first acute care admission to the health care system in over six years. Referral was made to Highland Hospital, and the patient was admitted through the attending MD on call. This admission lasted one week.

During this time, concerns were raised about finances. Did E.L. have the capacity to continue to provide care in the home? What resources were available to assist in discharge planning? Last, who would be the "backup" should home services be accepted? Those involved on the team included social service, attending MD/NP, family adult protective, home health service, and most importantly the patient. Her wishes to remain in her home were clear. Development of this care plan involved putting the CNC philosophy described in Figure 5 into practice.

Barriers that were met were lack of family/emergency backup. The client refused home services. At this point, it was arranged that a daughter who lived several miles away and worked full-time was willing to arrange a medication schedule and assist with the housekeeping. Those family members who lived in the next apartment were not willing to participate. Requiring home oxygen and frequent medical visits, it was agreed that the NP would make home visits to follow up and monitor her condition.

Case Study II: F.K. is a seventy-seven-year-old female patient from the SHS. Initial contact began with this patient on 12-05-91. The diagnoses at that time included obesity, emphysema, congestive heart failure (CHF), peripheral edema. This patient, due to morbid obesity, is confined to her home. The first visit in the home was for acute onset of shortness of breath and increased edema. At this time, it was decided to increase her diuretics and monitor for increased distress. Over the ensuing months, visits were primarily for acute

Figure 5 Client centered care.

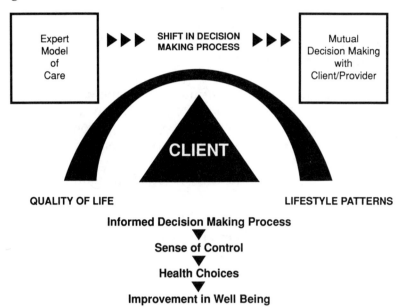

changes in respiratory status due to CHF which responded well to an increased dose of diuretics. Home visits were made on a monthly basis and as needed. This aggressive home follow-up is an example of tertiary prevention, because it prevented costly return to the hospital in a least four instances.

On 4-5-93, F.K. experienced extreme shortness of breath and chest pain. On the initial visit, it was felt that the patient needed to be evaluated in the emergency department. On physical examination, she had marked shortness of breath, was in moderate discomfort, and had significant increase in peripheral edema. Due to the patient's fear of acute admission, the family was called to lend additional support. The providers were able to arrange for the patient to be met in the emergency department by the provider. The patient was admitted and due to complications throughout her admission remained in the hospital approximately two months. The patient's admission occurred at a facility where the SHS was not affiliated, and thus the patient was followed by a different physician.

On her return home, she again contacted the SHS office requesting that the NP continue with home visits and coordinate her care with her new physician. The NP at the SHS office contacted her MD who agreed to continue a co-managed care relationship in the provision of primary and tertiary prevention for this patient. Her diagnoses remained the same. Plan for home care included the following:

1. Monthly house calls by the NP.
2. Home Health Aide approximately sixteen hours per day to assist with ADLs.
3. Visiting Nurse home visits every two weeks.
4. Physical therapy consult to assist with optimizing strength and mobility.
5. Dietary consult to reinforce 1500 calorie ADA diet to assist with weight loss.

This plan was developed through a case management conference held with her primary care MD and NP, Visiting Nurse, Home Health Aide, Family, Physical Therapy, Nutritionist, and most importantly the patient. The main goal was to optimize physical status in order to increase ADL tolerance.

Several acute home visits have been made due to the diagnosis of cellulitis and bronchitis. Hospitalization has been avoided through this aggressive team effort. The cost savings not only to the patient, but also the health care systems are significant. A future health services research goal in the CNC is to attempt to quantify and measure the cost savings of collaborative models of care such as the one described here. The overall benefit of this tertiary prevention approach has maintained the patient in her own environment, and has improved her quality of life and well being despite acute changes in her condition. This is an excellent example of the CNC philosophy of practice as evidenced in Figure 5.

The case studies presented above, depict another advantage of having a nurse-managed clinic such as the SHS and the benefits shared by those that utilize this practice. NPs are involved in many aspects of health care across the care continuum. The advantage of the provision of tertiary prevention is well described in the SHS practice and in these case studies. Not only are health care dollars saved, but clients are able to remain active partners in their health care and decisions surrounding their treatment.

The application of the Neuman Systems Model reiterates the importance of primary and tertiary prevention in health care. Through these prevention efforts, both NP and MD providers can decrease the cost of secondary prevention, acute care admissions, and emergency care. Collaborative efforts by the entire health care team can facilitate this paradigm shift from curing to a more holistic model of "caring."

FUTURE

The innovation and flexibility of this satellite faculty practice were key in the development of this collaborative practice. It serves as a model for both nurse practitioner students and community health students. Additionally, the joint clinical venture between a primary care residency program and the community nursing center has the opportunity to bring the role of the NP forward significantly in the context of health care reform. The focus of the adult nurse practitioner in collaborative practices such as the one in this chapter will be ongoing and continue to evoke and involve change.

Collaborative practices such as this one not only reinforce a holistic care model, but also facilitate expanding health care services to those with limited access. Mundinger (1994, p. 213) also believes that patients will be less litigious because "patients in those practices receive more comprehensive and satisfying care than they would be given in practices composed of physicians only or nurses only." There must be attention to the paradigm shift from curing to caring, especially for the populations served by practices like the Senior Health Service.

Although there will be obstacles whenever something new is developed, the benefits of such a unique, collaborative practice cannot be overlooked. The NP has the opportunity to become the "wise hero" as described by Walker (1993, p. 64), especially for chronically ill patients requiring primary and tertiary prevention. As the development of the University of Rochester's CNC continues and the role of the NP in health care reform becomes more dominant, collaborative practices such as the one described in this chapter will be the practice of tomorrow.

REFERENCES

Avorn, J., Everitt, D., & Baker, M. (1991). The neglected medical history and therapeutic choices for abdominal pain: A nationwide study of 799 physicians and nurses. *Archives of Internal Medicine, 151,* 694.

Bessman, A. (1974). Comparison of medical care in nurse clinician & physician clinics in medical school affiliated hospitals. *Journal of Chronic Disease, 27,* 15–125.

Brown, S., & Grimes, D. (1993). Nurse practitioners and certified nurse midwives. In *A meta-analysis of studies on nurses in primary care roles.* Washington, DC: American Nurses Publishing.

Charney, E., & Kitzman, H. (1971). The child health nurse (pediatric nurse practitioner) in private practice: A controlled trial. *The New England Journal of Medicine, 285,* 1353–1358.

Lewis, C., & Resnick, B. (1967). Nurse clinics and progressive ambulatory patient care. *The New England Journal of Medicine, 277,* 236–241.

McLaughlin, E., Anderson, E., Cesa, T., Larson, P., Johnson, H., Gibson, J., Lemans, M., & Delucchi, K. (1979). Nurse practitioners' public health nurses and physicians performance of clinical simulation test: COPD. *Western Journal of Nursing Research, 1,* 275–295.

Moccia, P. (1993). Nursing education in the public's trust—A faculty of the community: No unreal loyalties for us. *Nursing and Health Care, 14*(9), 472–474.

Mundinger, M. O. (1994). Sounding board—Advanced-practice nursing—Good medicine for physicians? *New England Journal of Medicine, 330*(3), 211–214.

Neuman, B. (1982). *The Neuman systems model,* 2nd ed. Norwalk, CN: Appleton-Century-Crofts.

Walker, P. H. (1993). Care of the chronically ill: Paradigm shifts & directions for the future. *Holistic Nurse Practice, 8,* 36–66.

10

Adolescent Care: Community-Based Faculty Practice in a Nursing Center

Donna Hill
Patricia Hinton Walker
Sue Groth
Nancy Chevalier
Adrienne Springer

Children and youth in America are growing up today in an environment that seems to encourage risk-taking rather than health-enhancing behavior.

Oda, 1991

A dolescent health care has challenged providers and the health care delivery system for decades. In an attempt to address issues related to inadequate access, complexity of care, and costs, new models for care of adolescents are being actively created by health care providers in an attempt to address the needs of this challenging population. " Adolescents are the only age group whose mortality rates have increased in the United States in the past 20 years" (Irwin & Millstein, 1986, p. 28). New federal initiatives such as school-based clinics and insurance reform are discussed frequently as a partial solution to providing services to this increasingly vulnerable population.

Recognizing the needs for adolescent care in community-based settings, the University of Rochester Community Nursing Center (CNC) has developed specific initiatives for advanced nursing practice with adolescents. This CNC has facilitated the development of innovative satellite faculty practices, many of them serving the adolescent populations in urban and rural settings. Benefits of this effort have been seen in: (a) an increase in access to and quality of care; (b) the early development of data bases; (c) an increase in knowledge and skill of faculty in understanding changing adolescent needs; and (d) exposure of students to developmentally appropriate nurse practitioner care and scholarly faculty practice. This chapter will describe faculty practice services designed for adolescent populations in Rochester, New York, and the surrounding areas through an innovative community nursing center. Issues related to care of the adolescents will be discussed with emphasis on the opportunities and new role(s) for advanced nurse practitioner in community-based settings.

UNIVERSITY OF ROCHESTER COMMUNITY NURSING CENTER

The University of Rochester CNC has been previously described in Chapter 5. As a "center without walls," the CNC provides direct and indirect services in rural, urban, and suburban settings within a 50-mile radius of Rochester, New York. These services were developed and organized into four clusters which are: Services for Life Transitions and Developmental Changes, Services for Longer Term Continuity of Care, Services for Life Altering Crisis, and Services for Organizations, Business, and Health Care Providers (Walker, 1991, p. 19). Services to adolescents are best described under the Services for Life Transitions and Developmental Changes (Figure 1).

The majority of the CNC satellite faculty practices provide services to underserved populations. Although some may not view adolescents as an underserved population, in a study on health care expenditure patterns for adolescents, "nearly one-fourth of children and adolescents under 18 years of age did not see a physician at all during the course of a year." Newacheck and McManus (1990, p. 133). In an effort to address the specific clinical and system issues that face providers of care to

Figure 1   Life transitions and development change.

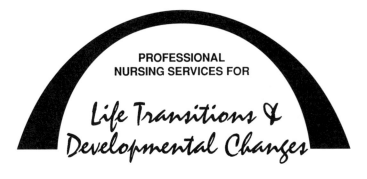

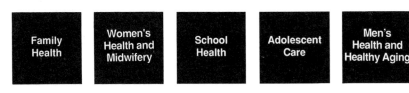

adolescents in upstate New York, the CNC has developed multi-service initiatives that build on the advanced nurse practi-tioner's (ANP's) base of leadership, initiative, and skill. They conduct service programs in a variety of sites designed to meet adolescents on their own turf. The use of ANP's also facilitates collection of data to measure outcomes and demonstrate the ef-fectiveness of new and creative ways to address current prob-lems in adolescent health care.

Using nurse practitioner clinical faculty members, the CNC provides access to care for adolescents and their parents/guardians through sites in medical clinics, schools, institutions,

Figure 2 Map of urban setting.

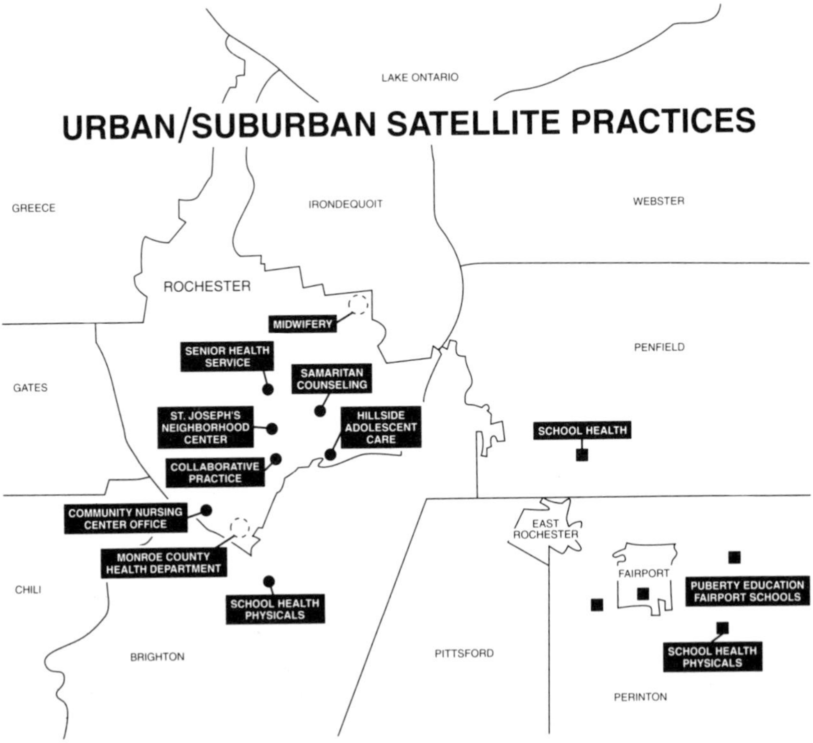

URBAN/SUBURBAN SATELLITE PRACTICES

and community-supported settings (Figure 2). Many of these services are directed toward the care of early, mid, and late adolescents. In addition to the benefits to the health care systems of the area, the programs supported by the CNC provide educational experiences for students in the University's schools of nursing and medicine.

The faculty and administration of the CNC are committed to exploring changes in health policy that will facilitate better care for this at-risk population. Recognizing that the key to serving adolescents and other vulnerable populations is to design truly community-sensitive practice, Community Nursing Center has developed an innovative and flexible approach. Rather than basing services on the strengths of individual faculty members, the CNC uses a matrix organizational structure to take advantage of diverse faculty practice skills and to create services that reflect client/organization-focused problem solving. This structure provides flexibility to meet the diverse needs of this population and supports development of a diverse resource of faculty practitioner expertise. Toffler (1990, p. 163), when discussing successful, futuristic organizations, coined the term "flex-firm." This type of organization must be networking in nature, with the ability to share resources, ideas, and data across product lines. Products (professional nursing services) and functions (of practitioners) may overlap, but this flexibility allows care to be provided to this diverse population in a variety of settings. CNC nurse practitioners providing care under this cluster of services include a school nurse practitioner, two pediatric practitioners, and a women's health practitioner.

With the organization structured as a "flex-firm," the CNC is prepared to develop new and diverse faculty practice services as community organizations present their needs. Women's health, pediatric, and school health nurse practitioners have the opportunity to share experiences, expertise, and practice patterns during monthly CNC meetings. In addition, two of the practitioners provide care at the county health department and have the opportunity to collaborate periodically. The women's health practitioner and a pediatric practitioner provide care at two different sites in group homes for troubled teens, and they periodically discuss similar cases and interventions as needed. During the peak times for conducting school health and camp physicals, the majority of these practitioners work together as a team to get the job accomplished in a variety of settings.

The faculty practices described in this chapter reflect the variety of ways that CNC faculty members interested in the adolescent population have worked to explore needs and propose programs that respond to the unique characteristics of various sites and populations (Table 1). A number of programs have been established and are flourishing in the community. The next priority is the development of an information system for data collection and measurement of outcomes of community-based care for this population required to influence health policy. Specific programs that describe CNC efforts to address the unique and challenging needs of adolescents in will be described in the following next sections of this chapter.

ADOLESCENT CARE AND ADVANCE PRACTICE NURSES

Generally, adolescence is defined as the period of transition from childhood to adulthood. There are wide variations in development of individuals throughout this time. Generally, care providers divide adolescence into three substages: early adolescence, middle adolescence, and late adolescence. There are differing classifications of these stages by age, which may be taken as evidence that the stages are best-defined by the characteristics typical of each. However, there are some issues that typify all of the stages.

Access to health care for these youths is complicated by many of the same issues that characterize adolescent development. The drive for increasing independence often means that adolescents want confidential care without parent or peer knowledge. The desire for normalcy and acquisition of identity require respect and genuineness on the part of care providers, despite

Table 1 Community nursing center sites for adolescents by service, adolescent age group, location, and numbers served/year.

Site	Service	Adolescent Age Group	Location	Number Served/Year
Canandaigua Medical Group	Primary Care	Early, mid-, late-	Rural	~500
Canandaigua Central School District	Sports Appraisals	Early, mid-, late-	Rural	~75
Fairport Central School District	Sports Appraisals	Early, mid-, late-	Suburban	~600
Fairport Central School District	Health Education	Early	Suburban	~650
Hillside Children's Center	Primary Care	Early, mid-, late-	Urban	~100
Hillside Children's Center—Satellite	Primary Care	Early, mid-	Urban	~100
Honeoye Central School District	Sports Appraisals	Early, mid-, late-	Rural	~50
Livingston Women's Health Clinic	Women's Health	Late	Rural	~100
Monroe County Health Dept.	School Care	Early, mid-, late-	Urban	~2,000
Penfield Central School District	Sports Appraisals	Early, mid-, late-	Suburban	~300

adolescent age-appropriate behaviors. Both peer pressure and the drive for independence mean that adolescents often are involved in high risk-taking behaviors, which require tact and high-level health counseling skills. Developing cognitive skills with variation in the ability to think abstractly means that care providers must be extremely skillful in communication and interviewing techniques specific to this age group. The increasing need for privacy, especially from families, mandates skill in negotiating resources, client advocacy, and counseling clients regarding their best interests. Finally, the adolescent's economic dependence on parents or guardians requires skillful accumulation of resources and negotiation with parents (McAnarney, Kreipe, Orr, & Comerci, 1992).

These same factors increase the likelihood that an adolescent will deny the teachings of health education and health promotion and will not seek care until there is a full-blown problem. They also contribute to the difficulty in arranging efficient and effective follow-up of medical and psychosocial problems. These unique characteristics of adolescents mean that care providers must be skilled in communication and interviewing techniques and be able to apply specialized knowledge about this age group to their practice. Often, physiological problems are accompanied by or caused by problematic behavioral practices. Thus, health care providers must have advanced knowledge of the physiological, developmental, psychological, sociocultural, and spiritual variables that may impinge on the adolescent's ability to maintain a healthy lifestyle.

Since time is needed to elicit specific information for an effective database and to compliment a diagnosis with health maintenance and health promotion activities, it is not fiscally responsible to have an adolescent seen consistently by a physician (Bibb, 1982; Brodie & Bancroft, 1982). The addition of advanced practice nurses to creative settings for health care has improved the quality of health care for this underserved population, while also addressing access and cost (Shoultz, Hatcher, & Hurrell, 1992).

The most visible evidence of the value of the ANP role in caring for this populations can be seen at Robert Wood Johnson School Health demonstration projects. In these efforts, school nurse practitioners have been placed in school-based or school-linked clinics. These sites have been successful in identification, treatment, management, and referral of adolescents. Yet to be solved are issues related to tracking of adolescents through the many potential sites of care; assignment of full-time primary care "homes" which adolescents will use consistently; and billing for service, because of confidentiality and adolescent's minimal independent income (Office of Disease Prevention and Health Promotion, 1993). These also affect the many specialty clinics that have been formed to address the needs of adolescents. However, these specialty clinics do not address many of the needs in the community. Community-based practices, such as those developed by CNC faculty to serve this population have more potential to reach adolescents where they live, than do specialty practices. The specific diverse services designed to meet the needs of this population are described in the next section of this chapter.

CNC SERVICES FOR ADOLESCENTS

School Health Services

The country has never before experienced the severity and complexity of health and behavioral problems in youth. Since the earliest trial of public health nurses in the schools of New York City at the turn of the century, nurses have used their knowledge and skill to respond to needs of school children and of the organizations that served them. The changes these nurses initiated have become institutionalized. For example, it is because of the public health school nurses' focus on prevention that we now have health educators and health education providing primary prevention curriculum in schools. Since schools have, most often, had the services of associate degree or baccalaureate nurses, it is an appropriate time to expose educators to the breadth and depth of advanced nursing practice.

In the first fall of the CNC's existence (1991), flyers were sent to all school district superintendents in the region. Then personal appointments were made with our contacts. In addition to working with communities and school districts to plan services, we have a variety of direct-service programs. The programs have been planned to meet the needs of the school districts and include primary, secondary, and tertiary prevention foci of care. Four components of the school health services that have flourished under the CNC umbrella: consultation services, school nurse practitioner services, school health physical examinations, and health teaching.

Consultation Services. Administrators easily connected CNC expertise with their needs. For example, after meeting with a local suburban district's administrator, the CNC was invited to conduct an organizational-process consultation and community assessment in order to help the school assume a proactive stance towards health services to meet the needs of adolescents in the twenty-first century. Parents, adolescents, school board members, administrators, teachers, support services, and pupil personnel services were involved in small group processing. The outcome of this effort was a report that provided guidance to the decision making by school administrators. The many organizational consultations of the CNC create opportunities for community-based consultation experiences for nursing students; a graduate nursing administration student was involved in the school effort.

School Nurse Practitioner Services. The Monroe County Health Department provides school health services in the city of Rochester. Through its school health programs, it supports a variety of services for adolescents, adolescent mothers and their babies, and adolescents in the workforce, as part of the school community. The problems of the adolescents in Rochester are typical of the profile of adolescents in any urban setting. In fact,

Rochester's rate of adolescent pregnancy exceeds that of New York City. The health department has contracted for the full-time services of an ANP who is a clinical faculty member of the CNC. Responsibilities of this position involve services to adolescents including:

- Entry and maintenance health appraisals;
- Athletic physical and work permit examinations;
- Exams for sexually transmitted diseases;
- Functional and mental health assessments;
- Coordination of follow-up care with physicians, other professionals, and other community agencies;
- Health counseling/health education for adolescents and parents; supervision of other nursing staff;
- Training/ resources to professional and paraprofessionals for staff development;
- Assistance with program policy planning, implementation, and evaluation;
- Consultation with education personnel in developing educational plans for children with special health care needs;
- Maintenance of records and reports.

This position provides faculty and nursing students with access to large numbers of adolescents from all socioeconomic groups and will provide data for future program planning and research. According to Oda (1991, p. 28) "investigations of the outcome of school nursing services are a high priority." In addition, the visibility of the CNC and it's potential for further initiatives is increased because, as part of her health department position, the faculty member will be a member of community and institution planning groups.

The competencies of advanced practice nursing are challenged by the variety of dimensions in the school nurse practitioners (SNP) practice. For example, in one week the school nurse practitioner (SNP) referred two students with previously undocumented heart murmurs and one with an enlarged, asymmetrical thyroid gland during a small work permit clinic. She also provided medical input in a meeting of school audiologists and technicians. In addition, a school nurse requested consultation about a contagious student and medical management of a student with herpetic lesions of the eye. The SNP provided liaison between the county health department's tuberculosis clinic and school health services regarding several students being directly observed for medication compliance. She worked to coordinate the efforts of the Foster Care Clinic (where another CNC clinical faculty provides care under a separate contract) with school health services. Another important function was the drafting of policies and procedures to expedite identification and management of tuberculosis throughout the school district.

The following case study illustrates the experiences with one of the adolescents who received care during the provision of school health services by the FNP. BG was an attractive, tall African-American who came to the Work Permit Clinic because she wanted "to find a job." Although her medical history and physical examinations were essentially negative, her psychosocial history indicated she had a "favorite" grandmother die in the past year. As the physical examination progressed, she showed little enthusiasm to questions about school, sports, her summer activities, or her plans for work. An expression of concern by the SNP that there didn't seem to be many "happy" things in her life resulted in her sharing that she had "problems" with her mother, no real friends, and little hope that it would get better. She had "thought about suicide" but had no plans or desire to end her life. However she didn't have any "energy" to help herself. With discussions, aided by the physical touch and distraction of the physical examination, she entered into a verbal contract to visit a local teen center for counseling. Follow-up was arranged with the school nurse and she managed a small smile as she left, referral materials in hand.

School Sports Examinations. Athletic physical examinations provide an opportunity for screening large numbers of adolescents each year. Schools have difficulty scheduling health care professionals to conduct these mass screenings each year. Two suburban and two rural school districts are provided with the services of ANPs through the CNC with the collaboration of the school physicians. At one of the suburban schools, there are mass, assembly-line screenings, whereas at the other suburban school there are individual, but large, scheduled screening clinics. The rural schools' sports physicals are conducted by school nurse-scheduled appointments. These screenings offer the opportunity to interview adolescents efficiently and find problems that require follow-up referrals. Schools find that CNC services are cost-effective, easily scheduled, and legally sound. The large numbers of adolescents who are screened by the nurse practitioners offer potential data for program planning and research.

Health Education. A large suburban school district had problems with their puberty education program and had discontinued its efforts. Consultation and collaboration with University personnel resulted in the development of a specialized educational program for early-adolescents in sixth grade regarding the changes of puberty with emphasis on providing facts to students and parents and encouraging families to assume responsibility for transferring information about values. Each year, CNC and medical personnel provide the program to approximately 600 students, and the program has now been moved to the fifth grade.

As a result of this initiative, CNC faculty and University of Rochester nursing and medical students have the opportunity to work with large numbers of healthy early-adolescents in a medically neutral environment. Among the University students, this has resulted in increased awareness of the requirements for anticipatory guidance at this stage in family development; development of skill communicating with early-adolescents and their families; and increased respect for the role of education and teachers in the life of these youth. The program also has potential for systematic study of this under-investigated population.

Institutions Serving Adolescents At-Risk

Institutions serving adolescents are challenged by the special needs of this age group, yet often have difficulties finding health care providers that are prepared specifically to work with these populations. For example, penal institutions have recognized that adolescents are vulnerable when placed in adult facilities and they appear to accept the rehabilitative and educational nature of incarceration of young people. However, responses to this age group are costly and time consuming. ANPs provide an alternative and effective source of specialized personnel for intervention with incarcerated or institutionalized youth.

Hillside Children's Center is a facility that serves troubled and emotionally disturbed children and families. It provides residential treatment, a campus school, day treatment, emergency shelter/crisis counseling, and therapeutic foster family care. The residential treatment facility provides care for 28 seriously mentally ill children and 14 hearing-impaired, mentally ill children requiring a therapeutic living environment. The emergency shelter offers emergency housing, crisis counseling, diagnostic assessment, and after-care services to children and families in crisis situations. The Juvenile Justice System tries to prevent permanent placement outside families by providing services to strengthen the family, but has a temporary penal program housed in a satellite facility of Hillside.

Nurse practitioner clinical faculty members from the CNC work in these three sites of the facility: the Hillside Residential site, Northhaven, and Appleton group home setting. Two nurse practitioners at these sites provide primary health care nursing services to at-risk female clients, group health care education programs, and individual health counseling. At the residential site, the practitioner frequently sees needy, troubled teens who come from troubled homes or foster care. These adolescent girls receive care at the Hillside health center from the CNC nurse practitioner during their stay in the residential facility. Often they have experienced sexual abuse and have psychiatric problems. One of the challenges with this population is to determine what is truth and what is fantasy. The girls are often involved in high-risk behavior and much of the practitioners time and skills are involved in physical examinations, diagnosis and treatment of gynecological conditions, and health education.

SU is a 15-year-old female resident at Hillside Children's Center. Her past history includes physical and sexual abuse by her father from age 7 to 12. She presently has problems with suicide ideation, self-abusive behavior, and a pattern of running away. SU frequently leaves the Hillside campus without permission and on these excursions is involved in sexual activity without protection. The CNC women's health nurse practitioner's contact with her began about 3 months ago as follow-up to her sexual activity. Interventions over the time period include: (1) physical exam with screening for STDs (sexually transmitted diseases); (2) education with frequent reinforcement regarding the importance of protecting herself from pregnancy and STDs; (3) education regarding available contraceptive options; and (4) education regarding choices and her right to choose to protect herself. At this time, SU has chosen a contraceptive method she feels will work for her. However, there is continued need to support her in making healthy decisions regarding her behavior.

Another CNC practitioner practices at the Northhaven and Appleton sites. Clients at the Northhaven are different from those at the residential site. Many of these adolescents have been picked up as PINS (Persons in Need of Supervision) by the police and are at Northhaven site for very short-term foster care. These adolescents will be placed in more permanent foster care, returned home, or sent to a treatment facility for substance abuse after a court hearing.

The majority of these adolescents are runaways, but they have not committed a crime. Approximately 99 percent are sexually active and usually at any given time at least 25 percent have sexually transmitted diseases. Only about 50 percent are using any birth control method and there are one to two girls between the ages of 12 and 16 that are pregnant in any given month. The challenge of care in this setting has to do with the very short length of stay. Only those adolescents where a pregnancy, STD, or other problem is suspected are referred to the nurse practitioner.

When the CNC pediatric nurse practitioner (PNP) first met YS, aged 13 years, she refused to let the nurse perform a pelvic examination "because she didn't need one." Her history included a previous case of gonorrhea, multiple sexual partners, no contraception, and intermittent lower abdominal pain. Her urine specimen showed 2+ leukocytes and a ph of 7. The PNP provided extensive individual counseling to impress upon her the need to take care of her body as well as reviewing the outcomes of untreated sexually transmitted diseases. After a discussion about the potential of having children and being a mother some time in the future, the practitioner described how advanced pelvic inflammatory disease could thwart that goal. YS returned to her temporary group home setting (with seven other girls) but she did return the following week for a pelvic examination. Results of her tests revealed that she had three sexually transmitted diseases. She was treated per CDC guidelines for gonorrhea, chlamydia, and trichomonas.

For the four or five weeks that she lived at the group home, she was also part of a one-hour, weekly discussion group run by this nurse practitioner author. Topics for discussion included physiology of normal maturation process, contraception, sexually transmitted diseases, peer relationships, and self-esteem building. YS was usually quite passive in these sessions, often seeming disinterested and bored. However, during her final week, before moving to a permanent placement site, YS was much more attentive, evidenced by her body language and increased participation. She began correcting erroneous statements made by some of the other girls related to the discussion. During that session, which was on the subject of sexually transmitted diseases, she said, very simply and definitively, "I'm not going to do that "stuff" (having sex) anymore right now. I want to be able to have kids someday." With this statement, this PNP author knew that something had changed for YS that day. At least at this point in time, this 13-year-old African-American girl was able to visualize a future goal and change her behavior to be more consistent with that goal.

The third site is a group home facility that is more like a home environment. Usually eight girls are housed in this facility and are selected because the social worker or nurse believe they could profit from this type of environment. The usual length of stay is about six to eight weeks. The CNC services provided at this site are educational in nature. The girls go to school on site, and one hour of class is taught that focuses on education related to sexual functioning and problems. Discussions relate to avoiding pregnancy, preventing STD and AIDS, and education about women's health issues. Also, special classes on adolescent skin care, relationship development, and self-esteem are provided. Although the girls are not at the home very long, there is time to help them think about new ways of approaching their transition into womanhood. No primary care is provided by the CNC practitioner at this site.

Physician and County Rural Health Care Clinics

Caught between childhood and adulthood, adolescents traditionally have been uncomfortably placed in adult internal medicine or pediatric practices. More recently, there has been an effort to create clinics specifically for this age group. However, many of the new initiatives, most notably school-based clinics, must provide access to a primary care provider, and sometimes this means that a pediatrician or internal medicine practitioner is ultimately responsible for the adolescent client's care. The medical community has responded to the needs of this unique population by creating adolescent specialists, but beyond the academic medical center, these specialists are in short supply. Thus, health care practices have initiated creative responses to provide specialized care by nurse practitioners having expertise with adolescent populations. One example of this type of practice is the CNC faculty practice within the Canandaigua Medical Group.

The Canandaigua rural practice is a collaborative practice with pediatricians of the Canandaigua Medical Group and consists of comprehensive primary care services for children from birth to 18 years of age. The facility hired a pediatric nurse practitioner who was interested in and capable of assuming leadership function with staff and for adolescent programming. In addition to her practice with children, the CNC nurse practitioner has developed specific service programs for adolescents at the clinic, and has precepted University graduate nursing students. Also, she provides consultation to school nurses in Canandaigua and Honeoye rural schools. Frequently, adolescents are seen for sports physicals in those schools. Addition of the specialized nurse practitioner in this rural setting has encouraged identification of health problems associated with adolescence, such as irregular or painful menses and stress-related syndromes. Common risk behaviors are discussed with all adolescents globally, with specific counseling as appropriate for individuals and families. The specialized expertise of this practitioner has increased awareness of the unique characteristics of adolescents by staff and families in this rural practice.

The following case study is typical of the adolescent clients seen in this practice by a CNC pediatric nurse practitioner who specializes in care of adolescents. BJ is a 14-year-old white female who lives at home with both parents, an 18-year-old sister and a 16-year-old sister. The 16-year-old sister was diagnosed with Ewings Sarcomas at age 4 and is considered a long-term survivor. In the past, BJ had a sledding accident and was treated for a Traumatic L5 Spondylolysis, Grade 1 Spondylolisthesis, Costo Chondritis, and is currently taking naprosyn as needed for pain. She has been seen in the pediatric offices in the past with a chief complaint of irregular menses. She described heavy to light flow on and off for five weeks, with no cramping, but stated that she had a loss of energy recently. She experienced menarche at 10 years of age, with regular once-a-month periods for approximately seven days with moderate flow. However, her menses had been irregular for 3 months after the sledding accident and surgery, then became regular again until 5/17/94. Last menstrual period started 5/17/94 with light flow and spotting, otherwise there was no recent illness or stressors, and no history of bleeding disorders. BJ denies sexual activity or abuse, denies smoking, alcohol, or other drugs. The clinical impression was dysfunctional uterine bleeding.

A CBC and Serum test were ordered and the lab results indicated CBC within normal limits and HCT = 36.8, pregnancy test negative. After discussing lab results with BJ and her mother, the practitioner prescribed O.N. 777 (28 day) 1 pill p.o. once a day as directed with two refills. In addition, Ferrous sulfate (325mg) for three months with interim support and teaching offered. Three months later BJ and her mother called stating that menses has been regular since starting OCPs. BJ had menses at the time of the call and was running out of OCPs. A prescription was called into the pharmacy, but the practitioner reinforced need for BJ to schedule an appointment within the next one to two weeks for further evaluation. Seven days later BJ was seen in the office. Her physical exam was unremarkable, with all finding within normal limits. At that time, the clinical impression was that menses were regular with OCPs, but she was still anemic. The practitioner's intervention was to continue the O.N. 777 as directed for three months, however this may be discontinued if menses continues to be regular for the next three months. Also, the Ferrous Sulfate was continued for one month with regular follow-up.

In Livingston County Health Department, Woman's Clinic, the faculty practice is staffed by two CNC nurse practitioners and serves clients at three rural sites. It is a county-supported health care clinic which was initiated in response to epidemiologic surveys and is staffed by a CNC women's health care nurse practitioner. This CNC practice was initiated by the needs of a rural county health department for nurse practitioners to provide preventive care. Since the main site is not too far south of Rochester, it was difficult for the county health department to recruit practitioners and compete with ANP salaries in the Rochester area. The health department director approached the CNC administrator, asking if there was some creative way that CNC clinical faculty practitioners could be brought to these rural sites to provide care. Since the CNC is established as a business model, it was impossible to provide care without adequate salary support for CNC practitioners. Consequently, a contract was negotiated to provide services at 80 percent time (or four days per week) by a CNC practitioner and another component of practice was built to complete the other 20 percent time of a full-time clinical faculty member (this 80 percent was based on the total amount of dollars available to the health department, which would only support 80 percent time including benefits). The nurse practitioner recruited happened to live in a rural community close to two of the Livingston county sites, so this arrangement met the financial needs of the practitioner, the CNC, and the practice needs in the community agency.

At a later time, due to the planned childbirth for the first practitioner, a job-sharing arrangement was designed with another part-time CNC nurse practitioner to meet the needs of this rural health department. These two practitioners continue to provide care at the three sites and their two part-time practices in this setting have served women and men in this rural community through health department clinics. Although this practice is considered a women's clinic, many of the clients are adolescents. Additionally, male clients (partners of women clients) are seen here by one of the CNC practitioners who has been trained to assist with diagnosis, treatment, and teaching related to sexually transmitted diseases. Although the primary practitioner is an adult practitioner, she has a keen interest and experience in care of women, and is equally competent caring for men's needs in this setting. These faculty practice sites have been used for precepting nurse practitioner students and is currently being used for nurse midwifery students as well. However, the location(s) sometimes create transportation and time problems for the students.

Community Agencies with Broader Missions

Communities are beginning to recognize their power to provide needed services locally and effectively. Opportunities for ANP interventions are beginning to open in churches, recreation/ community centers, and shelters. Adolescents are one of the chief concern of adults working to better the circumstances of their community. Thus, a mission of the CNC is to work with community groups to encourage specialized and competent services to their youth.

Sports Camp Physicals. The New York State Sports Camp for Adolescents is located in the city of Rochester and offers a summer sports camp experience for urban youth. A requirement of this program is that there be a health appraisal of the campers before acceptance. Teams of CNC ANPs journey to community recreation centers and schools to screen about 500 minority youth each year. They have been instrumental in augmenting the previously implemented minimum services and in adding a more complete health history. Follow-up services are provided by a camp nurse.

CONCLUSION

"Children and youth in America are growing up today in an environment that seems to encourage risk-taking rather than health enhancing behavior" (Oda, 1991, p. 28). Community nursing centers can contribute substantially to meeting the requirements for specialized health care of adolescents. Since this population is increasingly at risk and needs special attention from practitioners who are sensitive, yet competent to address the health promotion and prevention needs of this population. Moccia (1993) describes the need for the development of a "faculty of the community." Significant results of new efforts, such as those described in this chapter have the potential to impact of this advanced level and quality of care to this population; to improve access to care; influence health policy; and influence a shift in educational programming in the profession to nursing to the community. Community-based faculty practice, such as the satellite practices under the CNC umbrella at the University of Rochester are contributing in significant ways to the development of new and innovative practice roles, education of students, and research in the future, specifically in the area of adolescent care.

REFERENCES

Bibb, J. (1982). Comparing nurse practitioners and physicians on processes of care. *Evaluation and the Health Professions, 5,* 9–42.

Brodie, B., & Bancroft, B. (1982). A comparison of nurse practitioner and physician costs in a military outpatient facility. *Military Medicine, 147,* 1051–1053.

Irwin, C. E., & Millstein, S. G. (1986). Biopsychosocial correlates of risk-taking behaviors during adolescence. *Journal of Adolescent Health Care, 7*(6), 82S–92S.

McAnarney, E., Kreipe, R., Orr, D., & Comerci, G. (1992). *Textbook of adolescent medicine.*

Moccia, P. (1993). Nursing education in the public's trust—A faculty of the community: No unreal loyalties for us. *Nursing and Health Care, 14*(9), 472–474.

Newacheck, P. W., & McManus, M. A. (1990). Health care expenditure patterns for adolescents. *Journal of Adolescent Health Care, 11,* 133–140.

Oda, D. (1991). The invisible nursing practice. *Nursing Outlook, 39*(1), 26–29.

Office of Disease Prevention and Health Promotion. (1993). *School health: Findings from evaluated programs.* Washington, DC: U.S. Department of Health and Human Services.

Shoultz, J., Hatcher, P. A., & Hurrell, M. (1992). Growing edges of a new paradigm: The future of nursing in the health of the nation. *Nursing Outlook, 40*(2), 57–61.

Toffler, A. (1990). *Power shift* (p. 163). New York: Bantam.

Walker, P. H. (1991). The community nursing center for nurse practitioners, An opportunity to develop entrepreneurial skills. *Rochester nursing,* Fall, 19.

11

Reaching Out to the Working Poor: A Collaborative Effort

Phyllis J. Primas
Terri L. Mileham

We know how to intervene to reduce the rotten outcomes of adolescence and to help break the cycle that
reaches into succeeding generations. Unshackled from
the myth that nothing works, we can assure that children without hope today will have a real chance to become the contributing citizens of tomorrow.

Lisbeth B. Schorr

Nurses have a long and rich history of reaching and serving underserved populations. Therefore, it is not surprising that nurses are expected to be major players in health care reform, and that nursing's agenda for health care reform (Tri-Council for Nursing, 1991) has called for immediate action in the "nation's efforts to create a health care system that assures access, quality, and services at an affordable cost."

One of the largest groups of people with unmet health care needs is the "notch group," that is, families with incomes that fall below the Federal poverty level but above the eligibility level for Medicaid—largely our uninsured, working poor. Another group of currently underserved are those individuals in families where jobs, and consequently their health insurance, have been lost, but where other assets make them financially ineligible for assistance. Undocumented people living and working in this country comprise another large subgroup of the underserved.

In Arizona, children of the uninsured fare less well, in terms of both utilization of services and health status, than those insured by the Arizona Health Care Cost Containment System (AHCCCS, see appendix), the state's unique managed care program for Medicaid eligible clients (Flinn Foundation, 1989). Compounding the problem is the recent state legislation that disallows undocumented immigrants from AHCCCS eligibility. The only conditions for which services will be covered are emergencies and pregnancy (Dillenberg, 1994). Consequently, routine preventive and early treatment services are not provided for children in these families.

BREAKING THE CYCLE

One response to the need for providing services for uninsured children has been developed at Arizona State University, College of Nursing, as a component of a demonstration project of outreach primary care for children entitled "Breaking the Cycle of Disadvantage: A Nursing System of Health Care (Breaking the Cycle). Now entering its final year, Breaking the Cycle developed in response to increasing national, state, and local concern about the deplorable state of Arizona's one million children, as documented by the Children's Defense Fund (1990), the Governor's Office for Children (1990) and the Flinn Foundation (1989). The problem was further defined by the American Public Health Association in 1992, when Arizona was ranked near the bottom of the 50 states and the District of Columbia in access to medical care and a healthy environment. These reports presented a frightening picture of health care for Arizona children and support the literature that documents the relationship of poverty to both lower use of health services and poor health status (Call, 1989; Davis, 1991; Martin, 1992; Newacheck & Halfon, 1988; Pinkham, Casamassimo, & Levy, 1988; Rosenbach, 1989; Thompson & Hupp, 1992). Our existing health care system clearly had failed to reach those most in need.

Funding to initiate the project was obtained from the Arizona Department of Health Services (ADHS) in Fall 1990, with a renewable five-year contract. Due to the limited funding available from ADHS, and a desire to test our model of a nursing system of care in more than one target population, additional resources were needed. The principal investigator obtained a ASU Biomedical Research Support grant specifically for a pilot project to field test the methodology and feasibility of this nursing system in a small population of homeless children, prior to implementing the full demonstration. The Krause Memorial Children's Fund was established within the University Foundation, specifically to receive donations from individuals and organizations and to provide for needed services and supplies not covered by any other means. The county health department agreed to provide vaccines. The university entered into a service agreement with a low income school district specifically to provide health and developmental screening for high risk children as they enter preschool. Volunteer personnel were recruited to provide assistance at all clinics. The project has become a public/private/university collaborative endeavor.

Program planning and development of the outpatient primary care system included an extensive and comprehensive assessment of the primary care needs of children throughout the county. We applied a computer mapping technique to selected indicators so that we could determine geographic areas of priority. Following the identification of homeless children as the target population for the pilot project, we held a series of focus groups with parents of sheltered homeless children to obtain information relevant to meeting their needs.

A Community Advisory Board was formed that is comprised of state, county, and community leaders representing health and social services, children's advocacy groups, the religious community, education and housing, as well as multiple disciplines from within the University. Board members were selected for their commitment to improving children's health, their knowledge about existing systems serving children, and their agreement to participate actively in the planning, decision making, and evaluation of this project. A pediatrician, who has a long history of advocacy for mothers and children in Arizona, serves as the Board's chairperson.

An entire mini-health care system was developed specifically for this project. Portable clinic supply and equipment needs were determined and ordered, including a formulary of basic prescription medications. Financial and equipment donations were solicited. Personnel were recruited, interviewed, hired, and oriented. Policies, procedures, and protocols were developed, including a handbook to orient and assist clinic volunteers; volunteers were trained. Arrangements were made with a laboratory and with a group of consulting physicians. Client records were established, and the development of a computerized information system for use with lap top computers in the field, was initiated. A quality improvement system was developed. "Breaking the Cycle" was approved for state licensure as an out-patient treatment center on August 1, 1991.

The Model

The mission of Breaking the Cycle is two-fold:

1. To provide comprehensive, holistic, culturally acceptable and accessible outreach primary care services to selected populations of urban, underserved children and youth; and

2. To demonstrate the feasibility and cost-effectiveness of this unique mobile, "portable" nursing practice model of health care delivery." (Primas, Mileham, Toronto, & McCoy, 1994)

Conceptually, the model is based upon a defined, yet simple, philosophy: Children have a fundamental right to the opportunity to achieve their individual potential for health and well being. Multiple and interacting factors as defined by Blum (1983) (physical, social and economic environment, lifestyle attitudes and behaviors, inherited characteristics, and the health care system itself) need to be considered in planning for and in providing care to individuals, and families and communities. Consistent with Alpert (1988), our definition of primary care includes an approach to families as "the units of health and illness," and recognizes that there is an "inescapable social dimension to primary care services." We address the World Health Organization's (1978) definition of primary health care: "bringing health care as close as possible to where people live and work, and constitutes the first element of a continuing health care process."

We derived our title from the book by Liz Schorr: *Within Our Reach: Breaking the Cycle of Disadvantage* (1989). Based upon her careful examination of interventions that have worked for children and families in high risk environments, she concludes that effective programs will need to be more intensive, more comprehensive, and more flexible than traditional programs; as a result, they may also be more costly. Regardless of the sector being addressed (health, mental health, social services, or education), programs need to be able to respond to a wide variety of needs, reach out to locations where people live and congregate, and maintain staffs with the time and skill to establish relationships based on mutual trust and respect. She suggests that providing interventions in the health sector is a good place to begin, as such interventions also address a multitude of social problems. Our model includes the factors described by Schorr as being essential for successful programs.

There are three equally important and interacting dimensions to this nursing model:

1. Aggressive community outreach to identify children in need of health services;
2. The free, portable primary care clinic, which is provided in user friendly times and places; and
3. A referral and follow-up system to provide for continuity of care and to assist families in accessing services needed beyond the scope of the project." (Primas et al., 1994)

The entirely part-time staff includes a family nurse practitioner (FNP) who holds a master's degree in community health nursing and functions as the service director, a community health nurse (CHN), a health outreach specialist who is bilingual in English and Spanish, a research assistant who is university based, and an on-call consulting physician who is available by telephone. A pool of on-call pediatric nurse practitioners, family nurse practitioners, community health nurses, and Spanish speaking outreach specialists has been established to enable the project to readily expand into additional sites as supplementary funding permits.

Team members have multiple roles, functioning in both the clinic and the community. They are assisted by a cadre of volunteers, the project director, and a dentist who does the dental screening and assists in arranging for dental care. The team is available to reach out to the clients in their homes, schools, churches, shelters, or other places where they congregate. The emphasis, in all three service dimensions, is on health promotion, and prevention, early detection, and treatment of health problems.

Our service includes intensive outreach efforts to the target population by the health outreach specialist. Children in need are identified, often by other families or case workers, and encouraged to come into the clinic. Many parents hear of our services from others who have brought their children into a clinic. Since large numbers of our children are Hispanic, the outreach specialist's knowledge of the Hispanic community and skills in the Spanish language are essential for accuracy in translating materials from English, interpreting for other staff, communicating comfortably with clients and families in all settings, and developing an environment of mutual trust.

The outreach specialist is trained in prescreening for eligibility with the Arizona Health Care Cost Containment System (AHCCCS), Arizona's unique managed health care program for Medicaid eligible clients. She provides relevant health education (such as basic nutrition and hygiene skills, for which she has received additional training), and provides information related to available health, social service, education and legal resources for referral of children and their parents. Her responsibilities include assisting clients through the maze of the larger health and social service system as needed, and tracking and follow-up to ensure they have obtained necessary care. Coordination is developed and maintained with county Women, Infants and Children (WIC) workers, CHNs, other health and social service providers, and school and shelter personnel. In the clinics, the outreach specialist staffs the prescreening station, for which she has received the essential training, including state certification in hearing screening.

The benefit of outreach worker follow-up was clearly demonstrated in the following situation. A ten-year-old boy of American Indian decent presented to the clinic with severe dental decay, a swollen jaw, and obvious infection. His mother reported a history of similar problems in the past. Each time the boy would be kept home from school until he saw a practitioner.

He would be put on antibiotics, the pain and swelling would resolve, and he would be sent back to school without further treatment. The mother did not understand the need for additional follow-up nor did she have the resources to pursue treatment. Due to his background, he was eligible for Indian Health Services (IHS) and referral for urgent dental care was initiated by the Breaking the Cycle community health nurse. The outreach worker was assigned to contact the family and confirm that needed care was received. Several weeks later the child still had not been treated by a dentist. The mother had been unsuccessful in two visits to the IHS dental clinic due to system problems determining her son's eligibility. The local health department dental clinic was contacted and agreed to see this boy for his urgent dental needs. The outreach worker accompanied mother and child to the dentist and served as a liaison to the unfamiliar system and facilitated the completion of dental care that had been needed for months. Thus the boy was able to eat comfortably and return to school pain free.

The hub of Breaking the Cycle is the clinic itself. Supplies, including medications, are transported to each clinic from the project headquarters in the University's Community Services Center, in staff members' personal vehicles. The full service clinics are organized by stations through which children and parents flow and at which various aspects of service are carried out. The capability for a quick set-up of supplies has been developed for each station, and each staff member is responsible for bringing his or her station's supplies. Everything is or has been made portable, with the exception of scales, which remain at each site.

Whenever possible, on their first visit all children receive age-appropriate physical and developmental assessments according to the Medicaid Early Periodic Screening, Diagnosis and Treatment (EPSDT) guidelines. Additionally, all children, regardless of age, receive a separate dental/oral screening and oral hygiene education by a dentist; all children age one year and over receive a hemoglobin test; and all children who are mature enough to cooperate are screened for vision and hearing. Clients flow from the intake station, through the various screening stations, to the nurse practitioner, and finally to the CHN, who provides immunizations, makes referrals, and arrangements for follow-up, and provides a comprehensive, final review of the record before the child leaves the clinic. The numerous checkpoints facilitate the provision of necessary health education and important dialogue with parents and children.

When working with another agency, such as a school or shelter, Breaking the Cycle staff hold post-clinic conferences with agency staff to communicate regarding any problems identified, to help problem solve on the client's behalf, to expedite referrals and to arrange for any additional care needed. Children provided with medication and treatment may be given a return appointment for follow-up to determine treatment effectiveness, or scheduled for assistance from the outreach worker or CHN.

The FNP service director is responsible for the overall delivery of services and directly for the delivery of on-site clinical out-patient services. Her role includes physical examination of children, ordering of laboratory tests and treatments, prescribing and dispensing of medications to treat acute illness, age appropriate health education and counseling, consultation with physicians as needed, implementation of the quality improvement program, maintaining an adequate stock of medications at each clinic site, and recommending referral of children as indicated. She is available for consultation between clinics, as needed. Other responsibilities include obtaining evaluation data, and the orientation, training, and supervision of supplementary staff.

A unique pool position is that of clinical director. A family nurse practitioner (FNP) serves in this capacity. The primary purpose of this position is to maintain an updated, cost effective, basic formulary. Along with the consulting physician, the clinical director facilitates the provision of quality nurse practitioner services within the community standards of care by assisting in the development and revision of NP protocols and the evaluation of quality improvement activities. Hours worked per month vary depending on the need of the project.

The CHN is directly responsible for implementing and assuring the referral, follow-up, and coordination of services to clients. With consultation and input from other disciplines, the CHN trains, supervises, and supports the health outreach specialist who assists the CHN in her role. Responsibilities of the CHN/outreach specialist team are adapted from the nursing case manager model of service delivery (ANA, 1988; Maurin, 1990), and include:

1. Assessment of the need for services;
2. Planning;
3. Procurement, delivery, and coordination of services;
4. Monitoring to assure that the multiple service needs of the clients are met; and
5. Advocacy.

Goals of case management include the provision of comprehensive, quality health care, decreased fragmentation of care, enhancement of the quality of life, cost savings, and, ultimately, improved health outcomes. The CHN assumes case management in families with complex situations or children with special health problems, on a priority basis.

The Principal Investigator/Project Director (PD) maintains responsibility for the overall direction, management, and integrity of the project, provides liaison with College of Nursing, other university and community agency personnel, organizes and analyzes statistics, directs the record keeping and program evaluation components, determines new program directions, raises supplementary funds and manages the budget. She is assisted by the university-based research specialist. The PD also provides volunteer assistance at clinics by staffing the intake station, greeting, registering, interviewing, and orienting clients and parents, prioritizing children in need of service, orienting volunteers and visitors, and maintaining clinic flow. During the academic year, 20 percent of her faculty time is donated to the project by the College of Nursing.

THE TRINITY OUTREACH COMPONENT

During the first year of service delivery, the target population was comprised of homeless children in Phoenix, with services being provided in both the Salvation Army Family Shelter and the Trinity Episcopal Cathedral, which at that time housed a school for homeless children. As the population of homeless school children grew, the school was moved to another location. Meanwhile, individuals from the Cathedral, who were supportive of Breaking the Cycle and interested in developing an outreach health service, met with us to determine the feasibility of providing a clinic that would target underserved children in the community. Selected studies of outreach services to children have demonstrated their effectiveness in reaching populations in need (Goon & Berger, 1989; Jones & Nickerson, 1986). The church is located centrally to the two highest areas of geographic need identified in our project's initial needs assessment. It is also an ideal place for a clinic, as it is easily accessible by public transportation and provides an environment of caring and trust.

A pilot project was agreed on that would include ten clinics and the related services of outreach and follow-up, and would test the feasibility of utilizing our model at this site. A gift from Intergroup Healthcare Corporation, an Arizona-based health maintenance organization, provided us with the needed supplemental funding. Clinics were planned for twice a month, alternating between Wednesday afternoon and evenings, and Saturday, over a three-month period, to help us determine the best time for utilization by this population.

Outreach—Marketing Our Services

A current challenge to prevention-oriented health services is the ability to market these services effectively. Marketing has been defined as "a set of methods designed to reconcile the resources and production capacity of an organization with the needs and preferences of the consumers" (Dever, 1991). It is based on a theory of exchange, whereby an organization offers goods or services of value to someone who is willing to exchange them for something else of value, such as time or money. Where a public service is being provided, the anticipated exchange is found in the satisfaction of and appropriate utilization by consumers needing the service, and ultimately in the improved health status of society.

Our previously implemented needs assessment had served as a market analysis to identify target populations needing this health service. However, we needed to insure that the appropriate population was made aware of the clinic and that services were accurately promoted.

Flyers were developed by the staff in both English and Spanish (back to back). They advertised the Free Children's Health Clinic at Trinity Cathedral for uninsured, non-AHC-CCS children, and included dates and times as well as the types of care to be provided: vision, hearing and dental screening, complete physical examination, treatment of minor illnesses, immunizations, and health education. The printing costs were donated by a member of the congregation. A catchment area was defined surrounding the church, and flyers in the form of door hangers were distributed within this area by members of the project staff, church members and other volunteers, about ten days before the first clinic and again about mid-way through the series. Additional flyers were sent to selected health and social service agencies known or thought to be in contact with low income, uninsured populations of children, usually with a cover letter from the project director or other staff member. Flyers were also posted in restaurants, fast food establishments, churches and schools within the catchment area. The Cathedral placed a notice about the clinic in its bulletin, and included a call for volunteers to assist at the clinics.

Site and Services

At the Cathedral, the clinic was set up in the dining room, and children and their parents rotated through the six, clearly numbered stations. The nurse practitioner and CHN station were afforded privacy through the use of partitions that were donated by another church. To obtain a quiet place, the audiometer was set up around the corner in a room that otherwise serves as the church nursery. Signs were posted in front of the church and by the dining room entrance, so we could be found.

Since this was billed as a drop-in clinic, staff, and church members anxiously set up on the first day of the clinic to see if anyone would come. We were pleasantly surprised when seven clients appeared. Over the duration of this planned pilot, the numbers gradually increased to 28 and 30 children per clinic. As we spend a great deal of time with each child, it was obvious that more personnel were needed than originally planned; therefore, additional staff were assigned from our pool. As the large majority of these children were Hispanic, with monolingual Spanish speaking parents, additional Spanish speaking personnel were assigned to this clinic. Also, parents of some of the children were recruited to assist as volunteers, particularly to help with interpretation.

A unique feature at this site was the "play table," manned by a volunteer "play lady," who kept children occupied by assisting them with drawing, coloring or other games, while waiting between stations. Also, all children received a gift of toothpaste, brushes, and sugarless bubble gum from the dentist, following their dental education, and an age and child specific gift from the "Love Box," which had been donated by a kindergarten teacher and her class on Valentine's Day.

Findings and Evaluation to Date

The evaluation plan for this pilot project is the same as the evaluation plan for the total Breaking the Cycle Project, and includes the following components:

1. Attendance at the clinic and the identification of health problems;
2. Our ability to track children and identify positive outcomes;
3. Parent satisfaction with clinic services; and
4. A defined quality management program that incorporates internal and external record review.

During this pilot project, we provided services to 127 individual children in 177 clinic visits, plus numerous outreach home and telephone follow-up visits. An eleventh clinic was ultimately held in order to complete follow-up in return visits as necessary.We were clearly reaching and serving children in need. Preliminary descriptive analysis indicates that the most frequently occurring conditions at this site were dental caries and urgent dental needs, otitis media, anemia, and need for immunizations.

Criteria for "positive outcomes" were defined and evaluated as follows:

1. Children who were diagnosed as having otitis media (OM), provided with treatment, who returned to the clinic for follow-up and whose OM had resolved.

    Out of 20 children with OM, 15 (75 percent) were found to have a positive outcome. The remaining 5 did not return to clinic, and were not followed-up successfully.

2. Children who were found to be anemic, who either returned to clinic or whose hemoglobin was rechecked by the outreach specialist and found to be improving.

    Of the 18 children with low hemoglobin, according to Center for Disease control Standards, 12 children (67 percent) were rechecked and had a positive outcome. (One of the children not returning to clinic was found on follow-up to have gotten covered by private insurance.)

3. Children who were referred for specialist care—dental, visual, crippled children's services, speech evaluation, and other medical services, who were known to have had at least one visit for evaluation by the needed specialist.

Of the 41 children referred for specialist care at the time of this writing, only 10 children (24 percent) were known to have had a successful referral. Of the 41 children referred, 31 were referred for dental services; only 9 of these children actually received dental services; 6 of these 9 children had their dental services arranged by our volunteer dentist and paid for with specially designated monies from the Krause Foundation.

Response for lack of successful referral and follow-up include:

- Parent/guardian failed to follow-up;
- Limited time for outreach specialist to follow-up;
- Lost to follow-up; and
- Dearth of free or low cost resources.

Parent satisfaction with clinic services was determined by asking parents to complete a brief survey form evaluating the clinic. Our services were consistently rated "above normal" as compared to other clinics. Things parents stated they liked included the friendly and helpful staff, the time spent with each child, and the fact that we readily provided answers to their questions. Both the written evaluations and clinic attendance indicated no difference in preference between Wednesday evening and Saturday hours. Weaknesses of this evaluation include its selective nature—if the clinic was extremely busy, staff frequently forgot to ask parents to participate. Also, the clinic's environment was not conducive to maintaining anonymity; and the Spanish translation was not completed until services were well underway.

PHYLLIS J. PRIMAS & TERRI L. MILEHAM

While cumbersome and time consuming to implement effectively with a part-time staff, quality management chart audits were completed according to protocol, both internally by staff and externally by our consulting physician. Results and comments were compiled as group data and shared with staff.

Implications for Future

Because of the success of this pilot project, clinic staff and church representatives decided to seek additional funding to re-start and continue this service. To date, the on-going Trinity Outreach component has received additional gifts and grants from Intergroup Healthcare, Bank of America, Episcopal Human Services of Arizona, the Coalition for Human Needs of the National Episcopal Church, the Women of Valley Presbyterian Church, and other church and private individual donations. Significant sources of funding are needed in order to continue and expand this service, to include weekly clinics and additional sites, to add a needed psychosocial component, and to increase the ratio of outreach workers to client families.

While addressing our mission of public service, the location of the project in the College of Nursing provides rich opportunities for student clinical experiences and faculty practice. Selected community health nursing undergraduate students rotate through the clinic, identify client families, and provide interventions under faculty direction. Our nurse practitioners are being utilized as mentors for the increasing numbers of advanced practice students enrolling in the college's nursing program. The project also provides opportunities for faculty and student research as well as for employment opportunities, role modeling and mentoring of graduate students in all specialty areas. Expansion of our service base will, therefore, greatly expand our capability for providing student experiences with underserved populations.

The three dimensions of this model—community outreach, the primary care clinic, and follow-up—provide the basis for a comprehensive, holistic, community-based approach to reaching

REACHING OUT TO THE WORKING POOR

underserved populations. We are identifying and serving children who may not be reached in any other way. The model has the potential for replication and for expansion into other high-risk populations, and to include whole families and neighborhoods. It can be adapted to the needs of any given target population in a number of sites. The challenge remains to determine the most appropriate mechanism for integrating this model into the existing system of care.

In Arizona, certified nurse practitioners can practice independently, having a physician consultant available to them as needed. Our FNP/clinical director is listed on the clinic license as the "Medical Director." Nurse practitioners are also legally able to receive third-party reimbursement. Just recently, the legislature made it possible for them to serve as primary care providers within the various health plans providing managed care services to AHCCCS clients. We are in the process of applying for provider status for our nurse practitioners. However, within a totally managed care environment, nurse practitioner systems will need either to be included within existing health plans or to develop their own health plans, in order to provide the mandated twenty-four hour services. Interdisciplinary cooperation and collaboration will be essential to success. We believe this model of health care delivery is not only consistent with Nursing's Agenda (1991) but has the potential for making a significant contribution in response to the national call for *Healthy people 2000* (USDHHS, 1990) and the current efforts for health care reform. It demonstrates one effective mechanism for reaching many of our citizens who have the greatest need.

REFERENCES

Alpert, J. J. (1988). Primary health care for children and youth. In H. M. Wallace, G. Ryan, & A. C. Oglesby, (Eds.), *Maternal and child health practices*, (pp. 247–259). Oakland, CA: Third Party Publishing Co.

American Nurses Association. (1988). *Case management in nursing.* Kansas City, KS: Author.

American Public Health Association. (1992). *America's public health report card.* Washington, DC: Author.

Blum, H. L. (1983). *Expanding health care horizons.* Oakland, CA: Third Party Publishing Co.

Call, R. L. (1989). Effects of poverty on children's dental health. *Pediatrician, 16,* 200–206.

Children's Defense Fund. (1990). *Children 1990: A report card, briefing book and action primer.* Washington, DC: Author.

Davis, K. (1991). Inequality and access to health care. *The Millbank Quarterly, 69*(2), 254–273.

Dever, G. E. A. (1991). *Community health analysis: Global awareness at the local level.* Gaithersbury, MD: Aspen.

Dillenberg, J. (1994). *Public health and the undocumented immigrants: A discussion paper.* Unpublished paper, Arizona Department of Health Services.

Flinn Foundation. (1989). *Health care in Arizona: A profile.* Phoenix, AZ: Author.

Goon, J. M., & Berger, D. K. (1989). A model outreach program for health care screening. *Journal of Pediatric Health Care, 3*(b), 305–310.

Governor's Office for Children. (1990). *Arizona children . . . a special report.* Phoenix, AZ: Author.

Jones, E., & Nickerson, J. M. (1986). A time series study of the effectiveness and costs of EPSDT outreach in Maine. *Public Health Reports, 101*(1), 68–76.

Martin, D. A. (1992). Children in peril: A mandate for change in health care policies for low income children. *Family and Community Health, 15*(1), 75–90.

Maurin, J. T. (1990). Case management: Caring for psychiatric clients. *Journal of Psychosocial Nursing, 28*(7), 7–12.

Newacheck, P. W., & Halfon, N. (1988). Preventive care use by school-aged children: Differences by socio-economic status. *Pediatrics, 82*(3), 462–468.

Pinkham, J. R., Casamassimo, P. S., & Levy, S. M. (1988). Dentistry and the children of poverty. *Journal of Dentistry for Children*, January–February, 17–24.

Primas, P. J., Mileham, T., Toronto, C., & McCoy, B. J. (1994). Breaking the Cycle of disadvantage: A nursing system of health care. *Nursing and Health Care, 15*(1), 10–17.

Rosenbach, M. L. (1989). The impact of Medicaid on physician use by low-income children. *American Journal of Public Health, 79*(9), 1220–1226.

Schorr, L. B. (with Schorr, D.). (1989). *Within our reach: Breaking the cycle of disadvantage.* New York: Doubleday.

Thompson, T., & Hupp, S. C. (1992). *Saving children at risk: Poverty and disabilities.* Newbury Park: Sage.

Tri-Council for Nursing. (1991). *Nursing's agenda for health care reform.* Kansas City, MO: American Nurses Association.

U.S. Department of Health and Human Services. (1990). *Healthy people 2000: National health promotion and disease prevention objectives.* Washington, DC: Author.

World Health Organization/UNICEF. (1978). *Primary health care.* Geneva: Author.

APPENDIX

The Arizona Health Care Cost Containment System is Arizona's Medicaid program. It began October 1, 1982, as an experimental project after a fiscal crisis made it impossible for Arizona's counties to continue providing health care to the poor. Until that date, Arizona had no statewide system of providing health care to those in need.

While traditional Medicaid is "fee-for-service," AHCCCS is prepaid care. AHCCCS contracts with health plans in the private sector for the care of its members, paying them a predetermined amount each month for that care. This partnership between state government and private health plans is what makes the program experimental. No other Medicaid system in the country is run this way.

There are two major groups in the AHCCCS program: categoricals and state-funded-only members, made up largely of Medically Needy/Medically Indigent (MN/MIs). Categoricals are those people for whom AHCCCS receives federal matching funds. The MN/MIs are a state-funded-only population. People qualify for AHCCCS through the Department of Economic Security, the Social Security Administration, the various counties or through the AHCCCS long-term care offices. Once they are in the program, they receive the same medical benefits as everyone else regardless of how they qualified, with the exception of mental health services and some transplants.

Services available include doctor's office visits; hospital services; pregnancy care; specialist care; lab and X-ray services; medically necessary transportation; prescriptions; emergency dental and mental health care; mental health services for categorical children and young adults up to age 20, long-term care members age 65+ and the seriously mentally ill; medical supplies; and long-term care. Family planning services—but not abortion or abortion counseling—are also available.

AHCCCS is funded by federal, state, and county monies. The counties' contribution for medical services is fixed, but it varies for the long-term care program. Matching rates are negotiated annually with the federal government, and the rest of the budget comes from the state general fund.

In answer to the problem of the working uninsured, AHCCCS developed the Health Care Group, a small-business product that makes available affordable medical coverage to companies of 40 or fewer employees. HCG does not exclude any industries from coverage. The four benefit options available cover physician visits, hospital and surgical procedures, laboratory and X-ray services, prescriptions, and emergency care.

It is the goal of AHCCCS to develop an alternative health care delivery and payment system that contains costs and improves patient access while encouraging quality care. In March 1989, SRI International released a five-year study that showed AHCCCS was less expensive than traditional Medicaid and that AHCCCS quality of care was high. More recently, the Flinn Foundation in Phoenix released a study that painted a grim picture of health care in Arizona but said AHCCCS was meeting its goal of reaching the poorest of the poor. Another Flinn study showed that the overwhelming majority of AHCCCS members were satisfied with the care they were receiving.

As of August 1, 1994, the program had 464,718 members receiving care across Arizona. These people include pregnant women, children, physically and developmentally disabled, elderly, and families who previously had received care under the county system of health care. The program is in its twelfth year of operation and has been extended by the federal government until September 1994. Approval of an additional extension is anticipated.

12

A Nurse Managed Student Health Center— From Idea to Reality

Mary Jane Tranzillo

For every nurse practitioner, a practice that has grown so large and successful that you need to hire an extra physician.

Nursing Spectrum, May 1994

*C*ommunity Nursing Centers (CNCs) are organized, independent settings in which nurses function as administrators, supervisors, and health care providers and are accountable for all client care. CNC nursing staff perform health histories and physical examinations, diagnose and manage health-related alterations. Nursing staff work within protocols that delineate when consultation with a physician and/or referral is necessary. CNCs develop collaborative practice agreements with physicians who agree to provide consultation and to accept clients who are outside the nurse's scope of practice. The collaborating physician also reviews and signs the protocols.

CNCs may be free-standing or associated with an academic or service institution. The scope of services in a CNC includes management of minor acute and stable chronic illnesses; health maintenance/health restoration, including administration of immunizations, family planning, and functional assessment; health promotion/health education; and referral to other health care providers.

UMDNJ

UMDNJ is New Jersey's University of the Health Sciences providing education for medical, dental, nursing, basic sciences, and allied health professions students. The university has four academic health centers in Newark, Piscataway/New Brunswick, Stratford, and Camden, bringing health professions education to the entire state. The UMDNJ-SN Student Health Center (SN-SHC) provides services to students on the Newark campus.

The Newark campus of UMDNJ is located in a large urban community with a multicultural student population. Sixteen percent of the students are Asian; 13 percent are African American and .08 percent are Hispanic. Sixty-two percent of the students are over 25 years of age.

CNC

Need—Student Health

In 1991, the university approved a new policy on student health and immunizations. At the time the policy was implemented, students submitted their completed health records to their individual school. The records were then forwarded to another university in the state system with whom each school contracted to provide data entry services and compliance reports. Because compliance reports were not issued in a timely manner and health records were often lost, follow up on policy compliance became difficult and fragmented. The system, also based on the medical model, allowed for no emphasis on holistic health care or wellness.

The health and immunization policy, as revised in June 1993, requires students to obtain a health history and physical exam within six months prior to starting classes, a Mantoux test within three months prior to starting classes and annually, and evidence of having received the following immunizations: two doses of measles vaccine, at least one of which was given after 1980; one dose of rubella vaccine; one dose of mumps vaccine; diphtheria/tetanus booster within the last ten years; the three dose series of hepatitis vaccine and annual flu vaccine. The three dose series of polio vaccine is recommended but not required. Students are required to show immunity to varicella by providing either evidence of a medically documented case of chicken pox or serologic testing to determine the presence of varicella antibodies. Students may also meet the requirement for measles, mumps, rubella, and hepatitis by showing serologic evidence of immunity.

Collaboration

The deans of the schools on the Newark campus recognized the need for developing a mechanism to ensure student compliance with the new policy. The newly established (1992) UMDNJ-SN administration and nurse practitioner faculty saw an opportunity to meet this need and in spring 1992 began working with the Information Systems and Technology Department (IS&T) to develop computerized record keeping and reporting systems. Subsequently, the New Jersey Dental School (NJDS), the New Jersey Medical School (NJMS), the Graduate School for Biomedical Sciences (GSBS), and the School of Health Related Professions (SHRP) signed contracts with the UMDNJ-SN to provide review of each student's health record to assess compliance with university policy, to maintain the records, to enter the data in the Student Information System (SIS), and to issue timely summaries of student compliance to the associate dean of the appropriate school.

Center Development

In May 1992, UMDNJ-SN's coordinator for administrative and clinical affairs and the MSN program director saw an opportunity to develop a health assessment center where students could meet the requirements of the university's policy and receive affordable health care provided by nurse practitioners (NPs). Their discussions, which began with the concept of an immunization clinic open to nursing students and operating only during the summer months, quickly expanded into an NP-operated Health Assessment Center which would provide health histories, physical examinations, as well as immunizations, health teaching, and health promotion activities to all students on the Newark campus.

With the support of the UMDNJ-SN Dean and UMDNJ's associate vice president for academic affairs, space was negotiated in the Student-Employee Health Center, arrangements were made with a laboratory and radiology group, a fee structure was established, and brochures were printed and distributed to all of the schools. The medical director of Student-Employee Health agreed to act as the physician of protocol and standing protocols were developed in collaboration with him. The center, which opened in June 1992, was staffed by UMDNJ-SN faculty who contracted with the UMDNJ-SN to use the center as a faculty practice site. Financial support was provided by the UMDNJ-SN and UMDNJ's central administration in keeping with university's commitment to clinical practice.

Goals

The UMDNJ-SN SHC serves to enhance the health of the UMDNJ Newark campus student community by providing the necessary and appropriate high-quality preventive, diagnostic, and treatment services and to provide a clinical site for faculty practice and research. The SN-SHC has the following characteristics of a university wellness model: (1) preventive and educational health programs; (2) quality care; (3) cost effectiveness; and (4) active involvement in the local higher education community.

Staff

The SN-SHC is staffed by a director and advanced practice nurses all of whom hold full-time faculty positions in the UMDNJ-SN. Staff facilitators from the UMDNJ-SN Learning Resource Center also work in the SN-SHC. The SN-SHC provides students with an alternative health resource by complementing the services provided by the Student and Employee Health Services operated by the New Jersey Medical School.

Staff Activities/Responsibilities. The SN-SHC director is an adult nurse practitioner. She is responsible for planning and developing the SN-SHC, overall administration of the center, supervision of staff, and direct care of students. Planning and development activities include developing joint protocols in collaboration with the physician of protocol; reviewing and revising joint protocols as needed; developing the annual operating budget; and developing short and long-term strategic directions for the center. Administrative responsibilities include ensuring that an adequate inventory of biologics, stationary, forms, and medical supplies are on hand; scheduling staff; staff supervision and evaluation; contract negotiation with Associate Deans of NJMS, NJDS, GSBS and SHRP; coordinating data management services with personnel in IS&T; developing policies in collaboration with UMDNJ-SN administration and the physician of protocol; ensuring that expenditures are within budgetary limits; and preparing monthly reports for the associate dean for administrative and clinical affairs and an annual report for the SN dean.

Client responsibilities include reviewing all student records and evaluating them for policy compliance and alterations in health status which require follow-up; notifying the student, and, when appropriate, his or her associate dean, of areas in which follow-up is needed; entering all student data into the Student Information System; issuing compliance reports to the associate deans in a timely manner; providing direct patient care to students, including obtaining a health history, performing a physical examination, administering immunizations, health teaching and health promotion activities, and referrals for appropriate diagnostic studies or to the referral network and followup for stable chronic problems. The SN-SHC director serves on the University Student Health Services Advisory Committee as well as the Newark Campus subcommittee of this advisory committee.

The SN-SHC director reports to the UMDNJ-SN associate dean for administrative and clinical affairs. The SN-SHC director assumes overall responsibility for daily operation of the center and maintains close coordinating relationships with both the Newark Campus Deans Advisory Committee and the Students Advisory Committee.

All of the SN-SHC staff review health records with individual students, indicate areas of noncompliance and instruct students in the steps required to reach compliance. They also administer immunizations, perform health teaching and health promotion activities, and make appropriate referrals. In addition, NP staff perform health histories and physical examinations and clinical specialist/nursing educators refer students with minor acute health problems to the NPs for management. The referral network includes the physician of protocol, Student Mental Health Services, faculty in the Doctors Office Complex, dental school faculty, and Allied Health Professions faculty.

Hours of Service

The SN-SHC is open one day a week (Friday) during the fall and spring semesters. There is an answering machine which is checked daily so that inquiries can be addressed in a timely fashion. The SN-SHC director is also available by telephone and in person when not engaged in teaching activities in the UMDNJ-SN. During the summer semester, the SHC is open three days a week to accommodate the large volume of incoming and returning students.

The SN-SHC director acts as the staff NP during the fall and spring semesters. A clinical specialist and a nurse educator from the SN Learning Resource Center are also scheduled each Friday. Additional NPs are scheduled during the summer semester to accommodate the number of students who require health histories and physical examinations. Since many incoming students do not attend to the health and immunization requirements until the start of the fall semester, additional nursing staff are scheduled during the latter part of August. They assist with record review and administer immunizations.

Budget

The SN-SHC has three main sources of funding: contractual agreements between the SN and the other professional schools on the Newark campus, fees for service, and financial support from the UMDNJ-SN. Contractual agreements, as negotiated annually, call for the UMDNJ-SN to review and maintain student health records, enter the health data into the SIS system, issue compliance reports to the associate deans, and provide a mechanism through which students can receive the health services necessary to comply with the Health and Immunization policy.

Students who use the SN-SHC are charged on a fee-for-service basis, with a current fee for a history and physical exam set at $100. Immunization fees are based on the cost of the individual vaccine charged to the SN-SHC by pharmacy. There is an annual fee of $25 for record review and immunization administration, which is also designed to cover the recurring cost of medical and office supplies.

The UMDNJ-SN absorbed the start-up costs associated with opening the SN-SHC, including installation of sinks in each exam room, furnishing the waiting area and the exam rooms, obtaining file cabinets for student records, computer equipment, charges for computer lines to the AIS system, and a xerox machine. The UMDNJ-SN continues to absorb overhead costs, such as utilities and the director's salary, involved in operating the SHC.

Full-time UMDNJ-SN faculty are expected to engage in a nursing faculty practice as a regular component of their faculty workload. Several NP and clinical specialist faculty use the SN-SHC as a faculty practice site. Their salaries are paid from income generated by contracts and fees. The nurse educators from the UMDNJ-SN Learning Resource Center staff the SHC as part of their regular work assignment.

Analysis of SHC Services

The SN-SHC has been successful in improving student compliance with the university's Health and Immunization Policy. Because data is readily available, the associate dean of each school can readily exclude noncompliant students from class or clinical rotations until the health requirements are met. We have also been successful in identifying students who have never been given chemoprophylaxis for positive PPD reactions. These students are referred to UMDNJ's pulmonary center for further evaluation and treatment if indicated.

Health education and counseling has centered mainly on stress management, birth control, and safe sexual practices. We have also been effective in early detection of illness, including untreated urinary tract infections, unexplained hematuria, untreated anemias, and hypercholesterolemia. Recently, we identified a student with gross proteinuria and altered kidney function tests. These students are referred to their primary health care provider for further evaluation and are considered noncompliant with the health policy until they submit evidence of follow-up.

Research Opportunities

The SN-SHC is an area rich in opportunities for nursing research. Studies of student satisfaction with a nurse managed center, outcome studies of health care delivery, and attitudes toward NPs as health care providers, especially among medical students, are among the research areas open for study. The medical school has proposed a joint research project to study students who convert from negative to positive on Mantoux testing.

Future Plans

The UMDNJ-SN has submitted plans to UMDNJ's central administration proposing an expansion of SN-SHC services to include management of minor acute and stable chronic problems as well as a full range of women's health care services. This would require that the SN-SHC operate on a full-time basis. The proposal for a SHC administered via the School of Nursing has stimulated debate concerning scope of practice for advanced practice nurses, liability issues concerning joint protocols for management regimens, referral patterns within the university's medical community, perceptions regarding quality of care delivered by physicians versus advanced practice nurses, and questions of cost:benefit ratios. For example, some physicians have expressed the opinion that the care provided by nurse practitioners is inferior to that provided by physicians. Other physicians are reluctant to collaborate with nurse practitioners because of fears that in the event of a malpractice suit against the nurse practitioner they too would be liable.

As the concept of managed care and managed competition become realities, the health professions will increasingly see the benefits of working as an integrated team rather than as groups of competing services.

In 1994, UMDNJ formed a managed care corporation known as University Healthcare Corporation. Within this structure, local professional corporations were formed. The responsibilities of these autonomous units include development of regional health systems, development of primary care centers, and contracting with local managed care facilities to provide care and development of health product lines to be marketed to local managed care providers.

The UMDNJ-SN, together with the School of Health-Related Professions and the University Mental Health Services, has formed a professional corporation known as University Care Corporation (UCC). The purposes of UCC are to develop, provide, manufacture or market, products, technology, scientific information or health care services. At this time, the bylaws of UCC have been written and are awaiting final approval. In addition, the UMDNJ-SN is actively developing product lines. Under consideration are provisions for primary care services to family members of students at UMDNJ, establishing a home health service, and opening our primary care services to the community at large. This last possibility would allow the School of Nursing to develop a CNC which provides accessible, affordable health care to the medically underserved of the Newark community. We have identified 15 areas which must be considered as we plan for establishing a CNC:

1. Identify the population(s) to be served.
2. Establish a collaborative practice relationship with a physician of protocol.

3. Establish a referral network.
4. Establish a staffing pattern.
5. Determine the budget.
6. Establish reimbursement and billing mechanisms.
7. Establish hours of operation including how coverage will be provided during nonoperating hours.
8. Establish a system for medical records.
9. Develop protocols.
10. Determine the licensing and accrediting agency regulations which the health center must meet.
11. Write a mission statement.
12. Decide on a location.
13. Determine whether or not you are able to dispense medication samples and stock medications to patients.
14. Write job descriptions.
15. Establish total quality improvement parameters based on patient outcomes.

CONCLUSION

The idea of a SHC administered by the School of Nursing was formulated in response to the School of Nursing's need to monitor compliance with the university's Health and Immunization policy. The idea was marketed to the other schools on the Newark campus as a way to solve their problems of lost records and fragmented followup. The services provided by the SN-SHC encompass health teaching and health promotion activities which gives students an opportunity to receive wellness care. A proposal, which calls for an expansion of services to include management of minor acute and stable chronic health problems, has been submitted to the university's Central Administration. If approved, the SN-SHC would be an ideal setting for interdisciplinary education of students in all areas of health care. It would also provide opportunities for nursing faculty to carry out research in the area of health outcomes. In addition, the School of Nursing would be well positioned to become leaders in managed care at UMDNJ.

13

Advancing Nursing Centers within the Health Care Revolution: The Role of Research

Cecelia B. Scott
Linda Moneyham

There are seasons, in human affairs, of inward and out-
ward revolution, when new depths seem to be broken up
in the soul, when new wants are unfolded in multitudes,
and a new and undefined good is thirsted for. These are
periods when . . . to dare is the highest wisdom.

William Ellery Chandler, *The Union*, 1829

*T*he current movement toward health care reform is being propelled by a mood of impending crisis (Bridgers, 1992; Quindlen, 1994). A prevailing and widely accepted view is that the health care system is no longer effective in meeting the needs it was designed to address. Of particular concern are issues of accessibility, affordability, and accountability.

The impending crisis in health care and the movement toward reform are characteristics of a revolution in process. Kuhn (1970) noted that a crisis is a "necessary precondition for the emergence of something new" (p. 77). However, a crisis alone is not sufficient to bring about a revolution. The old does not give way until a viable alternative appears to replace it.

In the search for viable alternatives for reforming the health care system, advanced practice nursing has been promoted as one solution to the problems of accessibility, accountability, and affordability (Mikulencak, 1993; National League for Nursing, 1993; Schroeder, 1993). Moreover, the community-based nursing center, a model for the practice of advanced nursing, may well be the most revolutionary approach to health care to emerge from the profession. Nursing centers have received significant support within the profession, as demonstrated by the proliferation of nursing centers within the past decade (see Aydelotte & Gregory, 1989). It is estimated that, across the United States, 250 nursing centers are currently open for business (National League for Nursing, 1993).

Despite the profession's expectations and support for nursing centers, the revolution appears to have stalled based on a number of factors, including those often referred to as "irrational barriers"; namely, issues surrounding the legal scope of practice, reimbursement, and prescriptive authority (Pearson, 1993; Safriet, 1992). However, an important factor which is frequently overlooked is the paucity of research on nursing centers.

While many assertions have been made related to the value and effectiveness of community-based nursing centers, there is woefully little data to support these assertions. The potential contribution of nursing centers to health care reform cannot be effectively articulated until a number of issues have been addressed, including: (1) the identification of consumer needs, particularly those not being met by the current system; (2) a description of nursing interventions and their linkages with consumer needs and relevant health outcomes; (3) demonstrated effectiveness of nursing interventions in producing desired outcomes; and (4) demonstrated cost-effectiveness of services provided by nurses.

The role of research in the development of nursing centers must not be underestimated in addressing these issues. As Kuhn (1970) stated, "the decision to reject one paradigm is always simultaneously the decision to accept another, and the judgment leading to that decision involves the comparison of both paradigms with nature and with each other" (p. 78). Similarly, Bridgers (1992) argued that a necessary precondition for a true reform is a plan for demonstrating the effectiveness of any new model, particularly in terms of addressing consumer needs and issues of outcomes and costs.

While many nursing centers purport their aims include meeting the needs of consumers and conducting research to document effectiveness of the care provided, there is little evidence to support that such centers have actually reached their goals. Riesch (1990) and Lockhart (1994) noted that, in general, nursing centers are underutilized for research. Barger and Bridges (1990) noted that of 45 academic-based nursing centers surveyed, less than one research study per year was being conducted by associated students or faculty.

In making a shift from the old to a new paradigm in which nurses can play a major role, research must be undertaken to demonstrate the breakdown of the old paradigm and reveal meaningful components desired in the new system. Such research must demonstrate nursing's potential contributions. In this chapter, we will outline an agenda for generating meaningful data about nursing centers. In the following narrative, we will present an overview of extant research in order to identify critical areas requiring further research. Also, the data from a recent phenomenological study will be presented to: (1) reflect the value of qualitative inquiry as a starting place for defining the issues important to nursing as we position ourselves in health care reform; and (2) offer a tentative understanding of the value of a community-based nursing center from a consumer perspective.

OVERVIEW

The literature on nursing centers has focused primarily on description of the development and implementation of the nursing center concept (Barger, 1986a, 1986b, 1986c, 1991; Glanovsky & Provost, 1984; Hawkins, Igou, Johnson, & Utley, 1984; McEvoy & Vezina, 1986; Sharp, 1992). The earliest studies by Boettcher (1986) and Barger (1986b) focused on identifying and locating nursing centers. More recently, a small number of studies have focused on describing the characteristics of nursing centers, such as populations served and type of services offered (Barger & Bridges, 1990; Barger, Nugent, & Bridges, 1993; Higgs, 1989; National League for Nursing, 1993). Other studies have reported on the number of client visits, most common presenting problems, and client demographics (Foster & Moses, 1987; Grimes & Stamps, 1980; Hawkins, Igou, Johnson, & Utley, 1984; Hazard & Kemp, 1983; Newman, Sloss, & Andersen, 1984).

The NLN/Metropolitan Life study of nursing centers (National League for Nursing, 1993) was the first broad-scale study to attempt to characterize nursing centers. The study provided data about the clients, the financial status, and the major categories of services offered by such centers. Although this study provided a base for future studies of nursing centers, it generated little information for demonstrating the effectiveness of nursing centers in addressing the issues surrounding health care reform.

In a beginning attempt to demonstrate the effectiveness of nursing centers, a few studies have documented client satisfaction with the care they received in nursing centers (Bagwell, 1987; Gresham-Kenton & Wisby, 1987; McEvoy & Vezina, 1986).

However, the question that remains from these studies is what satisfaction with nursing care actually means. It is not clear what factors may influence client satisfaction ratings, nor is there a clear indication as to what they are satisfied with.

In-depth research which uncovers factors underlying a sense of satisfaction would be useful in identifying relevant interventions and outcomes and could do much in clarifying nursing's mission and purpose in regard to nursing centers. In addition, such data could be useful for identifying services valued by consumers and generating financial support for such services.

Conspicuously absent in the literature are studies which include the perspective of nursing center clients (Riesch, 1992). Such data is essential for documenting the gaps in services provided by the current health care system and the need for nursing services. Of particular importance is documentation that nurses provide services which are essential and cannot be provided by any other care giver. The perspective of the recipient of nursing care is a virtually untapped resource for identifying needs and problems of clients and the perceived value of nursing care in terms of providing needed interventions to produced desired outcomes.

The recipient of nursing care is a key source for documenting the value of nursing care and for assuring that nurses have a place at the table of health care reform. As a research method, qualitative inquiry can assist nurses, in partnership with their clients, to identify and more clearly articulate the elements necessary in determining the value and effectiveness of care provided within nursing centers (Schroeder, 1993; Scott & Moneyham, 1994). Consumer perspectives can provide insights into care issues not previously considered or underestimated by the provider as important in their influence on health.

Nursing's goals for nursing centers cannot be accomplished or supported without research. If nurses are to be taken seriously as contenders within health care reform, then we must provide documentation that nursing services are needed and produce quality outcomes which are cost-effective.

A RESEARCH EXAMPLE

The following data from a recent study demonstrates the value of qualitative inquiry in defining the issues important to nursing as we position ourselves in health care reform and a tentative understanding of the value of community-based nursing centers from a consumer perspective. In the study (Scott & Moneyham, 1994), we examined the perceptions and experiences of older adults using the services of an on-site, community-based nursing center. The nursing center was situated within a senior community of approximately 650 older adults and provided services via a nursing clinic, home visits, educational programs, screening programs, and care management.

Our phenomenological research design incorporated focus group methodology. Focus group participants were randomly selected from four major subgroups within and representing the community: (1) *Group 1*—community residents who served on the nursing center auxiliary and volunteered at the nursing center on a regular basis; (2) *Group 2*—community residents who had never used the services of the nursing center; (3) *Group 3*—community residents who had used the services of the nursing center on a regular basis during the previous six months; and (4) *Group 4*—community residents who had used the services in the past but who had not done so in the previous six months. The 27 participants ranged in age from 56 to 86, the majority (74%) were female, without a spouse (67%), and had a high school education or above (93%). Nearly half (44%) lived alone.

The findings from this study contribute to an understanding of consumer needs and the meaningfulness of nursing interventions as they influence client participation in health care, health outcomes, and cost-effectiveness. Although the major findings of the study are reported elsewhere (Scott & Moneyham, 1994), a number of other pertinent issues were derived from the data that have relevance to the present discussion. Two of these issues will be discussed here: (1) confronting the old paradigm; and (2) gaps in the old paradigm.

Confronting the Old Paradigm

It must be recognized that a shift in paradigm will necessitate a shift in consumer philosophy regarding health care, both in what constitutes that care and who provides it. The medical model of care is what is known to most consumers. The medical model supports and reinforces problem or crisis-oriented care, provided by and reimbursed to physicians. Confronting the old paradigm will be a challenge as nurses try to situate themselves as a major player within health care reform.

Consumer commitment to the medical model of care was evident in the study data, particularly in the group that had never used the nursing center services. For example, one participant stated, "Yes, I might come up [to the nursing center] if I felt like something was wrong and [the nurse] might tell me, 'Well you need to go to the doctor for that' . . ." Another stated, ". . . so I haven't taken advantage of many things [at the nursing center]. I haven't needed to, you know. But I think it is a wonderful thing to have here and I can understand that for people who have *serious problems,* that it would mean a lot to them."

These examples demonstrate both a problem orientation to health care and a lack of understanding of what nurses might be able to offer to health care consumers. Nurses have not been perceived to be in the forefront as primary care providers, but in a secondary position as assistants. In this regard, when no other provider is available, such as with low-income, vulnerable populations without choice, low-cost or free nursing services are frequently utilized. When consumers have a choice and are able to pay for that choice, it can be expected, as this data indicate, that the transition to nurses as primary care providers will be met with some confusion and resistance.

For instance, some participants who regularly used the nursing center viewed the services as valuable, but found themselves confronted by their medical care provider's concerns as noted in the following example:

My doctor knows that I come here [nursing center] for some things. At first he felt like maybe the government was interfering with the medical practice but I explained the situation here [nursing center]. And [the nurse] offered to send any resumes [forms] from my file and that pacified him.

Another participant stated it this way:

> Well doctors are very peculiar as you probably know. I have a friend of this area [senior community] who had blood pressure problems and her doctor told her he didn't want her coming here [nursing center] to have her blood pressure taken, he wanted to do it.

Participants' comments indicated that conflict or competition between their care providers was not useful to them. Rather, it created a sense of tension in their life. Conversely, participants frequently noted instances where the nurse collaborated with other care providers for their best interest. One participant described the collaboration this way:

> . . . in the beginning it [blood pressure] was up and there was no getting it down. One medication would bring it down, and two days later it would go back up again. Medication wasn't working. So the doctor knowing about [the nursing center] wanted to know if I thought the nurses here would be willing to take it at the same time every day, say for a week . . . and bring [the readings] back to him, which I did. And he immediately changed the medicine I was taking based on that . . . whereas it would have been difficult to have gotten to his office.

Another participant noted the importance of collaboration in addressing his wife's health concerns ". . . but my wife has [needed the nursing center]. Her doctor welcomed it . . . [the nurse] would do all these different things and so forth and she would call him [the doctor] and talk to him over the phone; naturally we appreciated that." Clients also related how the exchange of written information between providers was useful, as noted in this example, ". . . [the nurse] made me come back regularly while I was going to the doctor and they would tell the doctor in the meantime. They would keep a record and send that to the doctor. They would cooperate with him and I think that was good."

As nurses attempt to articulate their role in health care reform, due consideration must be given to the need for collaboration and exactly what form it will take. It is insufficient to suggest that collaboration is important and then make the banner argument that nursing can provide the same services as doctors at a lesser cost. In varying ways, participants in this study stated that they were not ready for a substitution, regardless of the value, but a call for collaboration between providers.

Consumers will play a major role as to whether nurses and nursing centers will be considered a viable force within health care reform. The nursing center concept, however, is not recognized or understood by the majority of the American public (Barger, 1985). This data further emphasizes the need to elicit consumer perspectives, assist consumers to identify and articulate the problems of the old paradigm, and delineate more precisely what nursing has to offer the public. A common sense approach to reform requires relevating the value and effectiveness of respective providers, avoiding duplication of services, and positively affecting the health of the client.

Gaps in the Old Paradigm

The current medical model of care prescribes a narrow role for nurses which is medically dependent and focused on problem-oriented, physical care. Moreover, morbidity and mortality are the outcomes of care traditionally used within this paradigm. Based on these measures, effectiveness of care avoids consideration of interventions or outcomes which are meaningful to the consumer or that delineate nursing's contribution to client health.

Our study findings, however, help to identify autonomous nursing interventions valued by the consumer and the concomitant outcomes related to health. Data generated from the study indicated that services deemed as necessary or desirable extended beyond traditional physical, illness-oriented care, and were not always available from physicians. Personal stories, as related by participants, suggested that having access to nursing services enhanced their sense of health and well-being. Access to care, psychosocial interventions, and environmental issues were among the many gaps identified in the old, medical paradigm which were being addressed by the nursing center. Each issue is discussed in the following.

Access Issues. Access is frequently defined in terms of resources to purchase health care. However, there are a number of other factors which influence access to care, even for those with adequate financial resources. Data from the study support this assertion on many different levels. For example, the inability of study participants to reach their physician served as a barrier in many situations. Having the nursing center available, on the other hand, provided the access perceived to be needed and affected the participants' sense of well-being. One participant caring for her ill husband relayed this story:

> After a few days I realized he was not responding to medication and that indeed he was far worse off than he was when he started [the medication]. So I called and talked with [the nurse] and she came to the apartment to see him because there was no way he could even walk. But anyhow, she took one look at him and immediately called his doctor and he advised that we take him off the medications immediately, which we did . . . and miracles do happen and within 48 hours, without a walker or anything, he was out walking and in the parking lot. I am convinced, had we not had a nurse to see him, because I could not get him to the doctor, I think the man would have died. He wanted to. I don't think we could live without it [nursing center].

For some participants, access was an issue due to the length of time and energy associated with getting to a doctor's office, as reflected in the following comments, "A lot of people feel too bad to go to the doctor, and you go and sit and sit, and wait. . . . I think in that case, they would rather they had home nursing." ". . . if you wake up and maybe your blood pressure is up . . . you don't want to make an appointment two weeks from the day." One participant stated emphatically:

> I don't think there's anybody here, if they were sick and had a choice between [the nurse] and doctor . . . I've heard many people say, and I would swear on a bible, I would rather, if [the nurse] could come to my house . . . I would trust her. I've seen her with people. I would trust her.

Participants' comments indicated that having nursing services available and accessible made the difference of whether they would seek needed assistance or not. In some cases, physician services were often used when nursing services may have been more appropriate and less costly. In other situations, the participants noted the importance of having the nurse available to assist in making the most appropriate decisions related to health care resources. For example, one participant reflected on her experience of having shortness of breath and feeling unsure of what to do:

> . . . I told her [the nurse] "I feel kind of strange and I don't know what it is. I am short of breath and when I was talking with you I felt that way" . . . . [the nurse] told me to call and get an appointment with the doctor and [I told the nurse] . . . my appointment's next week and she [the nurse] said "Well, that doesn't make any difference. You don't wait until next week. You go and call them and tell them you have to have an appointment before then." So she said, "If they give you any trouble I will call them on the phone and talk to them" . . . But I felt like I would not have existed if I had not gone to see about it and if she [the nurse] hadn't insisted that I do it.

Psychosocial Interventions. The data also indicated that services viewed as valuable by participants were not always available from their physicians. The need for psychosocial intervention (i.e., listening to concerns, support, or interpretation of information) was among the gaps frequently identified by group participants.

The importance of having someone listen or be available during times of concern is reflected in the following comment:

> You might not go to a doctor for grief counseling. . . . Like me, I came home and I was just burdened you know . . . but I didn't think about my doctor. . . . So I look and it was a day the [nursing center] was open, I called and they [the nurses] said come on down.

One participant, whose father was a doctor, summarized it this way, ". . . the [nurses] here have been very helpful. They are much more understanding than any doctor I have been to."

Being taking seriously when discussing their concerns was also noted as important:

> . . . just to be able to talk about it and have somebody to talk about it with, and nobody is going to down them for talking about it and no one is going to reprimand them and say "Ah, come on, you just think about this nice thing, and oh, you got grandkids." This is ridiculous when they come out with that.

Participants' noted that such interventions impacted on their sense of well-being. For example, one participant stated:

> I've been under a lot of stress lately. My mother is quite ill and I've had some problems with my husband's health. It kind of put a burden on me and I didn't realize it was creating stress. I came down here [nursing center] one day when I just felt like I just had to talk to somebody and saw one of the nurses and just kinda unloaded you know with her . . . and it did help relieve some of the stress.

The importance of specific and accurate information was also identified by participants as a factor influencing their well-being. However, under the medical paradigm, such information was not always forthcoming. For example, one participant stated: "Well, sometimes I think when you're dealing with these doctors, they're in such a hurry, you know, that they really don't take the time to tell you what's up." Conversely, nurses were viewed as an accessible resource for needed information: "You don't usually get the information [from the doctor] that you get from the nurses in the clinic. I think that it is a very special thing, really I do."

Stress has long been recognized as a factor affecting the health of individuals. However, interventions related to stress have received little attention from nursing or medicine unless a crisis becomes manifest. Participants in this study made clear that stress was operant in their lives and having someone knowledgeable to listen, provide support, and interpret complex information related to health and health care served to diminish their stress level. As noted in the data, nurses were viewed as a reliable and appropriate resource for this intervention.

Environmental Issues. Within the medical paradigm, health care is primarily focused on care as provided within institutions, without due consideration to consumer context or environment. However, the environment has long been recognized by nurses as one factor contributing to health. Providing services within the community where consumers live and work has enabled nurses to more fully incorporate this important factor.

Knowledge of and familiarity with the community and home environment provides data necessary for determining the most appropriate interventions to promote health and well-being. Assessment via observation, for example, was recognized as leading to an intervention facilitating comfort and functionality for clients:

Now if the nurses tell them (management) that they know that somebody has trouble getting up and down the steps, then a ramp is built almost immediately and I have seen the results of that on two occasions when the nurse just observed that someone had problems. Like next door to my apartment there is a lady . . . that the nurse upon visiting some in-house patients noticed the difficulty she had because of severe arthritis and they came and asked her if she wanted a ramp and it was built immediately.

Inquiry in conjunction with familiarity of the home environment assisted the nurse to formulate interventions related to injury prevention for the client and stress reduction for the spouse as noted below:

My husband was in the hospital for a certain length of time, already it had been 2^1/$_2$ months since he had a shower. I had to give him a bath in bed because there was no way he could stand up in a tub without falling. . . . The nurses suggested what I might buy for the bathroom [safety bars]. . . . to make it safer for him. Even though I had to buy them . . . she called and ordered them and they were delivered to me the same day. . . . It was taken care of in 48 hours. But it was all done by the clinic.

Finally, the data indicated that when nurses are considered an integral part of the community and have constant interaction with consumers of that community, they can influence health prevention and health promotion activities. As one participant stated:

They have so many screening things. So many cancer screenings, eye, ear, feet . . . we are fortunate to have those services so close . . . [the nurse] is constantly urging us to come to those screenings. I think a lot of us would just let them go by unless there was an emergency.

Failure to incorporate environmental issues into care essentially ignores an important component of health. Environmental considerations can strongly influence prevention, a major area of health care reform. Certainly, numerous opportunities exist for nurses within nursing centers to document their role in this area of care.

CONCLUSION

The nursing center provides the profession with a unique opportunity to demonstrate nursing's potential contribution to health care reform. What must be demonstrated is nursing's ability to provide services which: (1) are needed and wanted by consumers; (2) are not provided by the current health care system; (3) cannot be provided by any other care provider; and (4) produce desired outcomes for health. At issue here is whether or not nursing can produce the documentation needed to be a major player in the process of health care reform.

Nurses must consider which methods are most useful in generating meaningful data that will serve as a building block for future research needs. Research efforts must be focused toward methods most likely to reveal the factors relevant to health care reform and amenable to influence by nursing's contributions. Qualitative research methods, which incorporate the perspective of the consumer, are extremely useful in addressing these issues.

REFERENCES

Aydelotte, M. K., & Gregory, M. S. (1989). Nursing practice: Innovative models. In *Nursing centers: Meeting the demand for quality health care* (pp. 1–20). New York: National League for Nursing Press.

Bagwell, M. A. (1987). Client satisfaction with nursing center services. *Journal of Community Health Nursing, 4,* 29–42.

Barger, S. E. (1985). Nursing centers: Here today, gone tomorrow? In J. C. McCloskey & H. C. Grace (Eds.), *Current issues in nursing* (2nd ed.) (pp. 752–760). Boston: Blackwell Scientific.

Barger, S. E. (1986a). Academic nursing centers: A demographic profile. *Journal of Professional Nursing, 2,* 246–251.

Barger, S. E. (1986b). Nursing center: From concept to reality. *Journal of Community Health Nursing, 3,* 175–182.

Barger, S. E. (1986c). Academic nurse-managed centers: Issues of Implementation. *Family and Community Health, 9,* 12–22.

Barger, S. E. (1991). The nursing center: A model for rural nursing practice. *Nursing and Health Care, 12*(6), 290–294.

Barger, S. E., & Bridges, W. C. (1990). An assessment of academic nursing centers. *Nurse Educator, 15*(2), 31–36.

Barger, S. E., Nugent, K. E., & Bridges, W. C. (1993). Schools with nursing centers: A 5-year follow-up study. *Journal of Professional Nursing, 9,* 7–13.

Boettcher, J. M. H. (1986). A national overview of nurse-managed centers. Paper presented at the Third Biennial Conference on Nurse Managed Centers, Scottsdale, AZ.

Bridgers, W. F. (1992). *Health care reform: The dilemma and a pathway for the health care system.* St. Louis: GW Manning.

Foster, B. E., & Moses, R. K. (1987). Satellite clinics for elder health care. *Geriatric Nursing, 8,* 188–189.

Glanovsky, A. R., & Provost, M. B. (1984). The ELMS College Nursing Center: An independent setting for translating theory into practice. *Journal of Nursing Education,* 209–211.

Gresham-Kenton, L., & Wisby, M. (1987). Development and implementation of a nurse-managed health program: A problem oriented approach. *Journal of Ambulatory Care Management, 10,* 20–29.

Grimes, D., & Stamps, C. (1980). Meeting the health care needs of older adults through a community nursing center. *Nursing Administration Quarterly, 4*(3), 31–40.

Hawkins, J. W., Igou, J. F., Johnson, E. E., & Utley, Q. E. (1984). A nursing center for ambulatory, well older adults. *Nursing and Health Care, 5,* 208–212.

Hazard, M. P., & Kemp, R. E. (1983). Keeping the well-elderly well. *American Journal of Nursing,* 567–569.

Higgs, Z. R. (1989). Models of academic nurse-managed centers. In *Nursing centers: Meeting the demand for quality health care* (pp. 103–108). New York: National League for Nursing Press.

Kuhn, T. (1970). *The structure of scientific revolutions.* Chicago: The University of Chicago Press.

Lockhart, C. (1994). *Community nursing centers: An analysis of status and needs.* Paper presented at the National League for Nursing, Council for Nursing Centers Conference, Los Angeles, January 3, 1994.

McEvoy, M. D., & Vezina, M. (1986). The development of a nursing center on a college campus: Implications for the curriculum. *Journal of Advanced Nursing, 11,* 295–301.

Mikulencak, M. (1993). The 'graying of America'—changing what nurses need to know. *American Nurse, 25*(7), 1, 12.

National League for Nursing. (1993). A promising trend in the American health care scene: Findings from the Metropolitan Life Study of Nursing Centers. *Prism: The NLN Research and Policy Quarterly, 1,* 3–5.

Newman, J., Sloss, G. S., & Andersen, S. (1984). Evaluation of a health program. *Geriatric Nursing, 5,* 234–238.

Pearson, L. J. (1993). 1992–93 update: How each state stands on legislative issues affecting advanced practice nursing. *The Nurse Practitioner, 18*(1), 23–38.

Quindlen, A. (1994, June 1). The nurse paradigm. *The New York Times,* A15.

Riesch, S. K. (1990). A review of the state of the art of research on nursing centers. In NLN publication 41-2281, pp. 91–104.

Riesch, S. K. (1992). Nursing centers. *Annual Review of Nursing Research, 10,* 145–162.

Safriet, B. (1992). Health care dollars and regulatory sense: The role of advanced practice nursing. *Yale Journal of Regulations, 9*(2), 417–488.

Schroeder, C. (1993). Nursing's response to the crisis of access, costs, and quality in health care. *Advances in Nursing Science, 16,* 1–20.

Scott, C., & Moneyham, L. (1994). Perceptions of a community based nursing center by residents of a senior community. *IMAGE.*

Sharp, N. (1992). Community nursing centers coming of age. *Nursing Management, 23*(8), 18–20.

14

Patterns of Development in the Hispanic Immigrant/Poor Children from Birth to Five Years of Age

Lenoa Michelle Rios

Those who are fighting the battle of life at great odds may be strengthened and encouraged by little attentions that cost only a loving effort. To such the strong, helpful grasp of the hand by a true friend is worth more than gold or silver. Words of kindness are as welcome as the smiles of angels.

E. G. White, 1974

*W*hen I was given the opportunity of working full time for the UCLA School of Nursing Health Center, three factors influenced my decision. The first was the uniqueness of the job itself—to be practicing nursing in an independent role in a nurse-managed, ambulatory care setting. The second factor was the privilege of providing a service to those who would otherwise have no access to health care; and the third, most exciting factor for me was the predominantly Spanish-speaking population at the St. Francis Center site in downtown Los Angeles.

The UCLA School of Nursing Health Centers provide care to adults and children. Both of the Nursing Health Centers are licensed in the state of California as community clinics. The Union Rescue Mission site has been in operation on Skid Row in downtown Los Angeles since 1983. The St. Francis Center site opened in January of 1990 after moving from the day care center Para Los Niños on Skid Row where well-child care was provided once a month by a UCLA pediatric nurse practitioner faculty member (Stuart, 1994). The Health Center at the St. Francis center site then expanded their services to forty hours per week, and increased staffing to two family nurse practitioners.

Although I am a family nurse practitioner, most of my experience has been in pediatrics. As the practice developed at the St. Francis Center site, the majority of clients seen were children. Reasons for families seeking Health Center services were for immunizations, to have Women, Infant, Children (WIC) forms filled out, to have physical examinations for school entry, as well as the episodic childhood illnesses. The Health Center is an approved Child Health and Disability Prevention (CHDP) program site, which is a state-funded program. Through this program, all children under the age of eighteen who are from low-income families and have no other form of private insurance for health care are entitled to a complete history and physical examination including vision, hearing, and developmental screening as well as urine dipstick testing, hemoglobin or hematocrit, and blood lead levels. All of the clients seen in the Nursing Health Center qualify under the low-income status.

When I began working in the Nursing Health Center, the practice as well as the concept of nurse-managed health care delivery was new to this particular population. In the beginning, while establishing the practice, quite a bit of the educational information shared with the clients/families centered around the role of the NP and the importance of health maintenance/illness prevention. Counseling regarding normal growth and development, dental hygiene, safety, physical findings, and their implications formed a routine part of the health assessments. Since the NPs in the Nursing Health Centers determined the standards of their practice, the time needed to provide this quality of care was also decided by the NPs in any given situation. This ability to spend time with the clients based upon their individual needs resulted in increasing numbers of clients seeking health care services from the Nursing Health Center. Clients and family members also voiced their preference in coming to the Nursing Health Center rather than go to other health care facilities.

The developmental screening tool used by the author during well child examinations was the Spanish translation of the Denver Developmental Screening Tool (DDST). This tool was used for all the children from birth through six years of age. Initially, I approached the developmental screening with the assumption that all children follow a specific pattern of development in accordance with standardized developmental schedules unless the child has had some trauma or illness causing developmental delay. That there would be some minor individual variation was also accepted as an assumption. After performing approximately twenty-five well child examinations, I began to notice that there were two areas where the children were found to be developmentally delayed. In the birth to eighteen-month age range, the delay was in the gross motor area; and in the two- to five-year age range, the delay was in the language area. It was at this point that I began to question the previously held assumptions. Several questions came to mind as I continued to work with the population.

- What impact does poverty have on development?
- Is it possible that Hispanic cultural childrearing practices influence the child development?
- What impact, if any, does immigration have on child development?
- Is it possible that being exposed to Spanish and English simultaneously affects speech development?

This chapter addresses the patterns of infant motor development through eighteen months of age and language development in Hispanic immigrant/poor children between two and five years of age. The topics are presented in two sections. Section one focuses on infant motor development and section two on language development. Explanations and analyses are based on Pesznecker's (1984) Adaptational Model of Poverty (Berne, Dato, Mason, & Rafferty, 1990). (See Figure 1.)

GROSS MOTOR DEVELOPMENT

In their book *Encounters with Children: Pediatric Behavior and Development*, Dixon and Stein (1992) have presented a developmental model that incorporates an ongoing evaluation of the child's developmental history and environment. They state that development is a series of "spurts and lulls" rather than a "smooth continuum," and that the physical, social, language, and motor areas of development are all interrelated. Therefore, one cannot focus on only one aspect of development without obtaining a complete history of the child and the child's environment. In the process of development, one task has to be mastered before the individual can move on to the next task since the tasks build on each other. For example, infants must be able to support their upper bodies with their arms when placed in the prone position before they can learn to roll over. Before this action can take place, infants must have first mastered head/neck control.

Figure 1   Adaptational model of poverty. *Source:* Adapted from Elizabeth Pesznecker (1984), "The Poor: A Population at Risk," *Public Health Nursing,1*(4), 237–249.

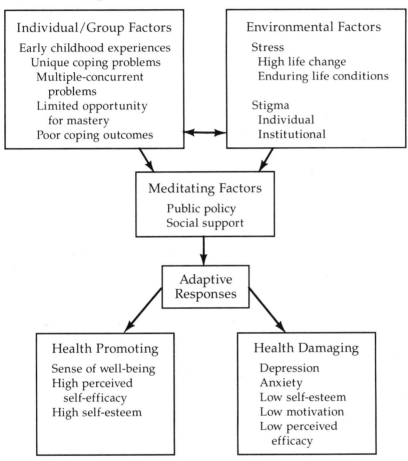

As previously mentioned, clinical observation must take place over time. All children are unique, have strengths and weaknesses as do their families, and have their patterns of development that are influenced by these factors as well as their culture, geographic location, and socioeconomic status (Dixon & Stein, 1992; Pesznecker, 1984). Nurse practitioners in a primary care setting are in an excellent position to provide this surveillance during well child examinations since the NP is the one who provides this ongoing care, is able to closely observe the child, has the established rapport with the child and the child's family, and therefore is able to provide early intervention when any deviations from the norm are noted.

The Master's prepared NP is educated to focus on broad health concerns with an emphasis on health promotion and disease prevention. Because of this focus, essential health care services provided by the NP include primary care interventions such as "health assessments, risk appraisal, health education and counseling, diagnosis and management of acute minor illnesses and injuries, and management of chronic conditions" (McCloskey & Grace, 1994, p. 22). It is in this context of the primary care setting, during these examinations/encounters which are performed by the NP, that the NP has the opportunity to gather the important data concerning the client, the client's environment, relationships, unique background, health beliefs/practices, observe patterns of development and other factors while establishing an ongoing relationship with the client and the client's family over time.

Developmental screening is a basic checklist of developmental milestones which one evaluates. It usually entails the application of a test to identify infants/children with a high possibility of having or developing a deficit (Lynn, 1987; Diamond, 1990). The tool should be sensitive, reliable, simple, fast, and easy to use (Greer, Bauchner, & Zuckerman, 1989). The tool that is most widely used and best known is the DDST and this is the one that was utilized in the clinic. The DDST is useful for screening children from birth to six years of age and has four major areas of developmental skills: personal-social, fine motor-adaptive, language, and gross motor. As outlined in the DDST, the areas of greatest developmental skills for infants is the gross motor and fine motor-adaptive. During the first year of life, infants should be developing muscle control and strength, that is, head/neck control, holding their chests up with their arms when on their stomachs, rolling over, sitting, standing, reaching for objects, bringing their hands together, and passing objects from hand to hand. With the exception of standing, all of the skills pertain to the upper body and extremities. From about ten to eighteen months of age, the focus becomes one of developing the lower body or extremities and culminates in the child's ability to walk well, stoop and recover, and negotiate steps.

In performing the DDST during the process of health assessment, I did not note any abnormalities from the first well child examination one or two weeks after birth through three months of age for infants who had a negative health history, that is, no birth trauma or illness such as meningitis, sepsis, or kernicterus. Beginning at about four months of age, I began to notice some developmental delays in the gross motor area, while there were not any notable delays in any of the other three areas. When placed on their stomachs, the infants were either not able to hold their chests up with their arms, or were unable to sustain the position for more than a few seconds. Furthermore, if kept in the prone position, the infants would begin to cry until they were turned over onto their backs or picked up. Older infants who were brought in for the first time and were screened could not sit without assistance or bear much weight when in the standing position. A review of the history and environment of these infants revealed the following factors:

- There is a general belief that it is not good for the infant to be in a sitting position or to leave the head/neck unsupported because the infant's spine may be damaged.

- The infant should not be placed in the prone position because the infant "doesn't like it" and "cries when placed in this position.

- The infant should not be placed in the prone position even when asleep because the infant might suffocate.

- The infant spends the majority of awake time in an infant seat or a walker.

- The parent or babysitter may have one or more other children that are toddlers and/or preschoolers and will leave the infant alone as long as the infant is quiet, therefore the infant may not receive much individual attention.
- Because of poor living conditions—roaches, rats, cold drafty floor, small quarters without much empty floor space; therefore, the parent/babysitter will not put the infant on the floor for fear of the infant getting hurt or becoming ill.
- Parental lack of experience and/or knowledge of growth and development.

According to Pesznecker's (1984) adaptational model of poverty, many of the above factors can be broken down into individual/group factors and environmental factors that can be attributed to the unique, complex problems of poverty. There is insufficient documentation in the literature relating to Hispanic childrearing practices to be able to establish this specific factor as an explanation for the slower gross motor development in this population. Pesznecker (1984) also states that the reactions of the poor to environmental stress and stigmatization are intrinsically involved in the process of coping, which in turn may be influenced by public policy and social support factors. How the individual/family responds to the interaction of all of the various factors will determine if the responses are "health promoting" or "health damaging."

Social support as defined by Kahn and Antonucci (1980) includes:

1. Affect—expressions of liking, admiration, respect, or love;
2. Affirmation—agreement, or acknowledgment of the appropriateness or rightness of some act or statement of another person and;
3. Aid—assistance given including things, money, information, time, and entitlements.

The role of social support has been documented in the nursing literature in various areas (Sisney, 1993; Brown, 1994; Jacob & Scandrett-Hibdon, 1994; Lewis & Brykczynski, 1994). That nurses have traditionally viewed their roles and functions more in the psychosocial area of "caring" versus the medical model of "curing" has also been documented (McCloskey & Grace, 1994). With the expanded role of the NP, both "caring" and "curing" interventions are necessary and are combined in the primary care setting of the Nursing Health Center with the primary focus being on the responses and needs of the client and the client's family as a whole (McCloskey & Grace, 1994).

In dealing with this particular Hispanic population, I felt that the infants and parents could best be influenced toward health-promoting behaviors through social support. The NP's social support intervention took the form of respecting the families and their cultural background, acknowledging their strengths by positively reinforcing initiation of well child visits and positive child care practices, providing information regarding specific games, exercises, and anticipatory guidance regarding growth and development at each clinic visit. These interactions resulted in adaptive responses leading to health-promoting behaviors. On subsequent visits, the infants were noted to be within normal limits as defined on the DDST.

LANGUAGE DEVELOPMENT

Language development is more complex than motor development and is not addressed in any substantive manner in nursing literature. Therefore, I borrowed from the areas of psychology and education in an attempt to explain this process within the clinical nursing setting. Whether language is the result of genetics or environment has long been debated (Brownlee, 1992). It is probably a combination of the two factors. It is accepted that all "human languages share certain fundamental structures and that children learn the complexities of language without being taught specific rules" (Brownlee, 1992). In her article "How many languages do you speak? An overview of bilingual education," Joan Erickson (1985, p. 8) states that "comprehension precedes production, and language is learned in context." Capute, Palmer, and Shapiro (1987) have said that language is the single best predictor of future cognition in the young child. And while prelinguistic skills of infants cannot predict later preschool language disorders or learning disabilities, studies have demonstrated a continuum from prelinguistic skills of infancy to the language skills of the preschool years. Preschool language disorders, however, have been known to indicate future learning disabilities. Recent studies in language development have not expanded on nor contradicted the preceding research.

Again, establishing a definitive explanation of the relationship between cognitive and linguistic development in preschool years is complex. According to Shonkoff (1992), some theorists have suggested that language and thought develop independently; others that language determines thought once a child passes beyond the sensorimotor period; and still others suggest that language and thought develop along parallel but independent pathways which merge after two years of age. Research on language development has been divided into four areas. Phonology analyzes the sounds in a given language. Syntax is the structure of the words or the rules of grammar. Semantics deals with the meaning and relationship of words. And pragmatics is the functional use of language; how questions are asked, how thoughts and feelings are communicated. It is the context.

Normal language development consists of two major milestones. The first is the receptive ability which involves the auditory alerting response. This is hearing and understanding what is said (Capute et al., 1987). This response is normally present at birth and is assessed on the DDST by ringing a bell and noting the infant's reaction. This action is also used to test the gross hearing of the toddler between one and three years of age. Children greater than three years are tested using an audiogram. Other receptive milestones include: social smile, responding appropriately to "no," waving bye-bye, and playing pat-a-cake as well as peekaboo, obeying a simple request or command without gesturing, and being able to point to named body parts. The second milestone is expressive ability. This ability consists of verbalization as demonstrated by cooing, babbling (vowel and vowel-consonant sounds respectively), single word usage (first without meaning and then with meaning), and immature and then mature jargoning. Expressive milestones can never be more advanced than receptive ones (Capute et al., 1987).

A pattern of delay in the language area was not as obvious as gross motor delay. As with the gross motor development, the initial findings in the language area of the DDST were essentially within normal limits up to about twenty months of age. The language tasks up to this age are vocalizing, laughing, the child turning toward the one speaking to the child, imitation speech sounds, and saying mama, dada, and papa. After twenty months of age, the language tasks become more complex. According to the DDST, there is a combining of hearing, understanding, and speaking. The child should be able to say three words other than mama and dada and point to one named body part before being expected to combine two words or to follow directions. Naming pictures, using plurals, giving his or her first and last name takes place between twenty-two and twenty-four months of age. All of the above come before comprehension of prepositions. The meaning of cold, tired, and hungry, and recognition of colors takes place next between three and a half and five years of age. The last three tasks outlined on the language section of the DDST include opposite analogies, definition of six to nine words, and describing the composition of a spoon, shoe, and door. No substitutes for these objects are allowed.

As already stated, becoming aware of any pattern of delay in the language area was more difficult because at this age, some children are shy, do not want to "perform on demand," and/or are anxious about the clinic procedures (e.g., Am I going to get a shot? What are you going to do to me? Are you going to hurt me?). Further complicating this scenario was the possible issue of bilingualism although the NP was not immediately aware of this aspect. It was only during the process of assessment and the establishment of rapport with the client and family that this awareness developed. On subsequent visits, a stronger bond was established and the client and family members were more at ease. Therefore, the children were more cooperative. After several months of administering DDSTs to these toddlers and preschool children in Spanish, I noticed that if the child was hesitant in naming a color or figure, and the child was not rushed or presented with another object, the child would sometimes answer correctly in English. The correct response was always positively reinforced by the NP. Since no specific guidelines are given regarding the scoring of correct answers in two languages when the DDST is used, the child was given credit for the correct response in either language. Because I had also had previous informal experiences with language development in other situations, her interest was intensified. This interest led me to more qualitative search of the literature on language development and bilingualism. This search revealed that those individuals who have studied the subject have done so in the form of individual cases, for example, by direct observation and description of family and/or friends' children, or small groups of monolingual and bilingual individuals. However, these research studies have, for the most part, not included toddlers and preschool children as subjects.

The following situations were observed by the NP. Included with the situations are possible explanations, supported by research, as to what may have been occurring in the child's language development. All of the families are Hispanic with Spanish being the primary language spoken in the home.

Situation 1. A two-year-old was presented with the DDST pictures. The child paused to look at each one of the pictures, but would not name any of them. When the father tried to coax her to say the word, he said "kitty." The child would not say the word, but was looking at the picture of the kitty. The

NP was surprised and asked the father if he was teaching the child English words for various objects. He answered "yes, some." Spanish is the spoken language in the home.

Situation 2. A two-and-a-half-year-old was presented with the pictures to name and without hesitation began to name the pictures; "gato," "birdie," "caballo," "dog," "un papa." The NP asked the mother if English was spoken at home and she responded "yes, sometimes a little."

Fred Genesee (1989) in his article "Early bilingual development: One language or two?" states that virtually all studies of infant bilingual development have found that bilingual children mix elements from their two languages. He also states that young bilingual children are psycholinguistically able to differentiate two languages from the earliest stages of bilingual development, and that they can use their two language systems differentially in contextually sensitive ways, thereby providing evidence of differentiated underlying language systems. In a study of 105 bilingual first graders, Umbel, Pearson, Fernandez, and Oller (1992) found that learning two languages simultaneously does not harm receptive language development in the language of origin while it does enhance performance in the majority language.

Situation 3. A twenty-three-month-old was presented with the pictures to name and named "gato" and "wow-wow." The child was given credit for saying "cat" but not "dog." If the child had only said "wow-wow," he would not have received credit and would have failed this particular task. It should be noted that the word "perro" (dog) is more difficult for a child of this age to say in Spanish, whereas in English, dog is easy for a child to say and is monosyllabic. The double "r" sound comes later in Spanish language development. Spanish was spoken in the home.

Situation 4. A four-and-one-half-year-old was asked to name the colored blocks. The child did not respond and became anxious, looking around, playing with the blocks. After completing the remainder of the examination, the NP again presented the child with the colored blocks and asked the child if he could name the color of the block held in the NP's hand. Again there was some hesitancy and anxious behavior. Finally, the child said falteringly "blue." The child was positively reinforced for giving a correct answer and the next block was held up. When the child didn't respond, the NP said in Spanish that he could say the word in English, and then repeated the same phrase in English. The child gave the correct answer in English. The child was able to name all four colors correctly in English. The entire testing had taken place in Spanish, since the child responded better when spoken to in Spanish, even though his answers for colors were in English. Spanish was the spoken language in the home. Although no English was spoken at home, the child was attending a day care center where English was spoken.

Lindholm and Padilla (1978), in "Language mixing in bilingual children," reported that when phrasal mixing occurred, nouns were the most frequently mixed lexical items. Structural consistency of the utterances was maintained so that there were no lexical redundancies or syntactic errors. It is possible that bilingual children mix words or phrases because they have heard mixed words/phrases spoken by their parents or other speakers in their environment. Mixed utterances are reportedly more frequent in the early stages of bilingual development and diminish with age. A study conducted by Naomi Goodz (1989) suggests that children's early language mixing does not reflect interlinguistic confusion, but rather that the child is formulating hypotheses about language based on the available data. Similarly, Francois Grosjean (1989, p. 6) in his article "Neurolinguists, beware! The bilingual is not two monolinguals in one person," states that ". . . the bilingual is an integrated whole which cannot easily be decomposed into two separate parts. . . . The coexistence and constant interaction of the two languages in the bilingual has produced a different but complete linguistic entity." He also declares that the individual who speaks two or more languages may have a third system in which the languages are combined. The use of the languages, either separately or together, is influenced by the needs of the individual, the environment, and interactions with others. The study by Umbel et al., (1992) concurs with the preceding two studies. Umbel et al., (1992) further states that when assessing a bilingual child's cognitive functioning based on lexical knowledge, "one must look beyond performance in either language to a union of skills in the two languages" (p. 1019).

Situation 5. A four-and-one-half-year-old did not answer when asked what the child did when the child was hungry, tired, or cold. The child also did not know the colors. The child came from a single parent family. The mother worked approximately twelve hours a day and the child was with the babysitter all day. The mother was also unable to read or write in Spanish or English. The babysitter spoke only Spanish and also cared for other children. On certain occasions, it was noted that the child was not dressed appropriately for the cool weather, even though the clothes she was wearing were always clean and pressed. If there is not enough money for food and appropriate clothing, the child may be hungry but not eat when hungry, or be cold and have no sweater or jacket. Therefore, the child may not be able to associate food with hunger or a sweater with cold weather.

Based on the above situations and many similar situations, I began to wonder how much of the "language delay" that was seen initially was due to poor stimulation because of poverty and all that it brings, and how much of the "delay" was the result of exposure to a bilingual environment. In all of the situations, the parents were immigrants. Some of the children had been born in a Latin American country, and some had been born in the United States.

Seeing these situations also brought to mind other personal experiences of children and their language development which depicted more environmental influences. A German family with a three-year-old child was living in Mexico. The child was able to converse fluently with his parents in German, fluently in English with other English-speaking missionary families, and fluently in Spanish with the local people. The level of conversation was typical of a three-year-old. As another example, my first niece was born in Mexico and lived there until she was six months old at which time her parents moved back to the United States. She mixed Spanish and English when she began to talk. Her sister was born three years later in the United States and could neither speak nor understand Spanish. The last example concerns an English-speaking friend who moved to Puerto Rico when her daughter was two years old. The daughter speaks Spanish and English fluently. Nine years later, this friend had another daughter in Puerto Rico who mixed both English and Spanish when she began to speak. When the second child was three years old, the friend had a third daughter who "wouldn't speak" at two years of age. Wondering why the child would not speak, the friend began trying various tactics and discovered that the child responded only when spoken to in Spanish.

The educational level of the parents in all of the personal examples was college or higher and the families were above the poverty level. In the clinic population, the level of parental education ranged from illiteracy to completion of college. All of the families who came to the clinic however, were at or below the poverty level. A review of the history and environment of these families revealed the following factors:

The child was exposed to varying degrees of English in conjunction with Spanish daily;

The level of parental/caretaker education was variable, therefore, stimulation of language development in either language was variable;

The physical needs of the child were possibly not met adequately nor in a timely manner;

The lack of access to educational materials in Spanish due to lack of funds and availability;

The lack of knowledge of bilingual development.

According to Pesznecker's adaptational model of poverty (1984), the above factors are integrated in the individual/group and environmental factors. The adaptive responses could lead to health damaging behaviors. Because of the child's diminished receptive and expressive language abilities due to the factors of poverty as well as the social stigma of being "different," that is, speaking a language other than the language of the country in which the child lives, it is important that the mediating factors be positive. Thus, the adaptive responses would then lead to health promoting behaviors.

Positive mediating factors that would lead to health promoting behaviors can be found in both the area of public policy and social support. Although the public policies in California relate more to the school-aged child, there are preschool programs available in both Spanish and English if the child meets the State requirements. If a problem is suspected in the area of cognitive and/or language development, an early intervention program is available through the State preschool program. Aspects of social support took the form of testing knowledge in both English and Spanish, positively reinforcing a correct answer in either language, not labeling a child "delayed" on the basis of one screening performance, initiating parent education regarding bilingual language development during well child examinations when the child is in the "babbling" stages of language development, encouraging parents to have the child's older school-aged siblings borrow library books in both Spanish and English and read aloud to the younger child, suggesting that the parent/caretaker watch the television program "Sesame Street" in either Spanish or English (both programs have segments in the "other" language), and encouraging parents to improve their language abilities. Resources for becoming literate in Spanish, if they were not, were provided as well as resources to learn English, if they desired.

CONCLUSION

The nurse practitioner in the Nursing Health Center setting is in an ideal position to provide the "caring" and "curing" interventions, ongoing surveillance, and social support which are fundamental for healthy outcomes. While carrying out these interventions, the NP is in a unique role because of his or her educational background, with its emphasis on health promotion and disease prevention. The child must be evaluated based on a knowledge of the whole picture. Care also needs to be taken not to label a child as developmentally delayed after only one screening examination. Labels have a tendency to stay with a person. Also, the primary health care provider needs to be aware that language development must be evaluated through the total language repertoire, as it is used in the child's everyday life, if one is to obtain a correct assessment (whether or not one is mono- or bilingual). What at first may appear to be an abnormality, may in fact be a strength leading to healthy behaviors/outcomes if positive mediating factors are a part of the practitioner's intervention. Positive mediating factors can be the result of well-directed public policy, as evidenced by the state preschool programs and bilingual education programs. Since there are no programs specifically directed at enhancing motor and cognitive development of infants, toddlers or preschool children under age four, the NP in the Nursing Health Center has the opportunity and responsibility of providing this testing, education and encouragement that these children/ families need to promote health. The effectiveness of the outcomes is enhanced by the NP's distinctive position as a primary health care provider in a Nursing Health Center.

REFERENCE

Berne, A. S., Dato, C., Mason, D. J., & Rafferty, M. (1990). A nursing model for addressing the health needs of homeless families. *IMAGE: Journal of Nursing Scholarship, 22,* 8–13.

Brown, S. J. (1994). Communication strategies used by an expert nurse. *Clinical Nursing Research, 3,* 43–56.

Brownlee, S. (1992). The southpaw's secret semantics. *U.S. News & World Report, 112,* 66.

Capute, A. J., Palmer, F. B., & Shapiro, B. K. (1987). Using language to track development. *Patient Care, 22,* 60–71.

Diamond, K. E. (1990). Effectiveness of the Revised Denver Developmental Screening Test in identifying children at risk for learning problems. *Journal of Educational Research, 83,* 152–157.

Dixon, S. D., & Stein, M. T. (1992). *Encounters with children: Pediatric behavior and development* (2nd ed.). St. Louis: Mosby Year Book.

Erickson, J. G. (1985). How many languages do you speak? An overview of bilingual education. *Topics in Language Disorders, 5,* 1–14.

Genesee, F. (1989). Early bilingual development: One language or two? *Journal of Child Language, 16,* 161–179.

Goodz, N. S. (1989). Parental language mixing in bilingual families. *Infant Mental Health Journal, 10,* 25–44.

Greer, S., Bauchner, H., & Zuckerman, B. (1989). The Denver developmental screening test: How good is its predictive validity? *Developmental Medicine and Child Neurology, 31,* 774–781.

Grosjean, F. (1989). Neurolinguists, beware! The bilingual is not two monolinguals in one person. *Brain and Language, 36,* 3–15.

Jacob, S. R., & Scandrett-Hibdon, S. (1994). Mothers grieving the death of a child: Case reports of maternal grief. *The Nurse Practitioner: The American Journal of Primary Health Care, 19,* 60–65.

Kahn, R. L., & Antonucci, T. C. (1980). Convoys over the life course: Attachment, roles and social support. *Life-Span Development and Behavior, 3,* 253–285.

Lewis, P. H., & Brykczynski, K. A. (1994). Practical Knowledge and competencies of the healing role of the nurse practitioner. *Journal of the American Academy of Nurse Practitioners, 6,* 207–213.

Lynn, M. R. (1987). Update: Denver developmental screening test. *Journal of Pediatric Nursing, 2,* 348–351.

McCloskey, J., & Grace, H. K. (1994). *Current issues in nursing* (4th ed.). St. Louis: Mosby.

Pesznecker, B. L. (1984). The poor: A population at risk. *Public Health Nursing, 1* (4), 237–249.

Shonkoff, J. P. (1992). Preschool. In M. D. Levine, W. B. Carey, & A. C. Crocker (Eds.), *Developmental-Behavioral pediatrics* (2nd ed.), (pp. 39–47). Philadelphia: W.B. Saunders.

Sisney, K. F. (1993). The relationship between social support and depression in recovering chemically dependent nurses. *IMAGE: Journal of Nursing Scholarship, 25,* 107–112.

Stuart, I. M. (1994). UCLA School of Nursing Health Center. *Connections, 3,* 1, 4.

Umbel, V. M., Pearson, B. Z., Fernandez, M. C., & Oller, D. K. (1992). Measuring bilingual children's receptive vocabularies. *Child Development, 63,* 1012–1020.

15

The Use of Health Risk Appraisal in a Nursing Center: Costs and Benefits

Thomas Mackey
Jeanette Adams

If I had known I was going to live this long, I would have taken better care of myself.

Unknown

*H*ealth promotion and disease prevention remain impor-tant concepts in all of the health care reform proposals debated in Congress. Nursing centers, which use nurse practitioners as principle primary care providers, focus on these very concepts. In fact, the delivery of health promotion and disease prevention programs has been identified as a predominant feature of nursing centers. In 1992, the American Association of Colleges of Nursing determined the primary reasons for the establishment of 62 nursing centers throughout the United States (Table 1). Meeting identified community needs, as well as providing avenues for primary care clinical experiences for both students and faculty, have been priorities. Reasons for operating a nursing center include: service, education, and research endeavors within a University setting; community care; care of special populations such as the homeless and indigent; delivery of primary care services to the population in general including health promotion activities.

This chapter describes one program of health promotion conducted in a nurse practitioner managed clinic—the use of health risk appraisal. The results of a research study conducted in an employee health service using health risk appraisal data, including the health-related and financial outcomes of the program, and implications for advanced nurses providing primary care in nursing centers is also discussed.

Using the worksite as a location for health maintenance and health promotion services is relatively new. Traditional worksite

Table 1   Reasons for establishment of 62 nurse clinics/centers.

Most Important Reason for Establishment	Number of Clinics	Percent
Community need	25	43.1
Clinical training site	23	39.7
Faculty practice site	7	12.1
Research site	2	3.4
Other reason	1	1.7
Not reported	1	

health programs focused on health and safety issues related only to the workplace. However, the occupational health community has increasingly recognized that individual lifestyle choices impact the worksite, both in performance effects and health costs of unhealthy lifestyles. The thrust toward promoting wellness and making the best use of human resources, through worksite programs, is becoming a common theme in occupational health (Anderson & Anderson, 1991).

Two important components in planning for health promotion and disease prevention programs are assessment of wellness and assessment of risk. For health promotion, Travis and Callander (1990) describe six categories of well being that can be evaluated on a continuum: physical, social, emotional, intellectual, occupational, and spiritual. The assessment of the level on a scale of well being can identify for the individual a need for more, or less, emphasis in a particular area. Assessment of wellness actually becomes a client's self-measurement and indicates direction for activity related to health-seeking behaviors.

On the other hand, risk assessment is designed to provide an awareness of how current behaviors and physical health measurements impact health. Methods of assessing individual risks include obtaining a health history, performing a physical examination, and obtaining specific laboratory data related to cholesterol, liver function, glucose, and other values.

HEALTH RISK APPRAISAL

Another method of evaluating health risks is to have patients self-administer a health risk appraisal (HRA). Health risk appraisals are used to measure modifiable and nonmodifiable health risks in a person's life. These self-administered questionnaires address the areas of well being (e.g., eating/nutrition, caring for self/others), fitness, environmental safety, personal habits, stress, responsibility, and attitudes regarding health.

HRAs are an important component of many occupational health programs, assessing and suggesting lifestyle modifications that workers can adopt to improve their health status (Warner, Wickizer, Wolfe, Schildroth, & Samuelson, 1988). Information gathered includes biometric data (height, weight, blood pressure readings, cholesterol levels), behavioral practices (smoking status, exercise, alcohol use, nutrition, etc.), attitudes towards health and health behavior, and other related information such as family and social history. These HRAs function as personal risk assessments and are used frequently to provide baseline data for planning health promotion activities and health education (Anderson & Anderson, 1991).

Although widely used, the effectiveness of HRAs for initiating and sustaining health-related behavior change has not been adequately documented. Their usefulness in educating workers and in promoting decision making regarding lifestyle changes has been proposed. Potential for cost savings to employers in terms of illness prevention has frequently been the impetus for implementing worksite HRA as a component of general health services. Frequently programs have been implemented without an evaluation component. As a result, the data has not been available and further research in this area is needed.

One obstacle to evaluating the use of health risk appraisal is the lack of documented reliability and validity for most of the instruments. The number of these instruments has increased dramatically over the last few years. The information from HRAs can statistically determine the odds that a person with certain characteristics and health practices has of developing disease or dying. Issues related to reliability and validity center around the accuracy of these statistical predictions. Expert input and review, using national data from population databases, has been used to develop recognized tools. The Carter Center instrument, the Life series of instruments, and others are based on the first generation of health risk appraisals, originally developed by the Centers for Disease Control (Society of Prospective Medicine, 1992). Validity has been reported based on review of the items by experts in the various health disciplines. Content validity has been established in that the items included are descriptive of health behaviors that are believed to be related to the risk of disease and death (Smith, McKinlay, & McKinlay, 1991).

A primary consideration regarding reliability is consistency of the information given by the individual. An individual's report of health history and health behaviors is, in the vast majority of cases, thought to be consistent enough to enable accurate calculation of risk (Smith, McKinlay, & McKinlay, 1989; Elias & Dunton, 1980). Reliability of the instrument is questioned only when the changes in participant's response would change the risk calculation. In a study of 338 adults aged 25 to 65 years, test-retest reliability was calculated on an HRA given 7 to 12 weeks apart. The areas of family history, smoking, and weight were reported consistently ($r > .75$), but lifestyle and physiologic parameters were less stable (Smith et al., 1989). In another study, test-retest reliability for a group of 25 men who completed HRAs at a time interval of 3 to 5 days ranged from .75 to .99 (Alexy, 1984).

The Life Survey instrument by Wellsource (1989) was chosen for use in the nursing center based on availability and computer support for analysis in another component of the health science center. This tool contains 219 items, including demographic information, nutrition, health habits, safety, and health-related attitudes. A risk analysis is computer-generated and includes scores in fitness, stress/coping, nutrition, safety, wellness attitude, and number of health practices. The overall wellness score is a statistical determination based on the weighted subscores. The information on the number of health practices is based on longitudinal research by Breslow and Enstrom (1980) who reported that there were selected health behaviors associated with positive health status and longevity. Seven habits were identified: avoidance of tobacco, regular exercise, eating breakfast, adequate rest (7 to 8 hours of sleep per night), regular meals with limited snacking, no or moderate alcohol intake, and weight in the recommended range for height. Those who identified six or more of the health habits were shown to live 12.5 years longer than those who reported three or less, and had a better health status.

IMPLEMENTING HRA IN A WORKSITE HEALTH PROGRAM

In September 1992, the University of Texas Nursing Services-Houston (UTNS-H) began to service the contract for delivery of employee health services at the University of Texas Houston Health Science Center. Prior to that time, the Department of Family and Community Medicine provided these services along with other primary care services to the community.

UTNS-H is a nurse practitioner directed clinic providing primary care services. As such, UTNS-H emphasizes primary prevention and health education, in addition to other primary care services. In agreeing to provide the university with services to employees, it was a priority that primary prevention services would be established as part of routine care in the clinic. At present, the most significant and widely used primary prevention approach is the provision of health risk appraisal. In the period September 1992 to August 1993, 418 new employees of the pool of 847 new hires voluntarily participated in health risk appraisal, representing 52 percent participation.

After hire, but prior to actually beginning employment, all new employees are required to complete a health screening examination at the nursing clinic. Part of the screening examination includes the opportunity to participate in health risk appraisal (Life Survey by Wellsource). On the day of the employee's appointment, a history, physical assessment, and laboratory examination is completed. Testing for tuberculosis is done using the Mantoux test. The employee is given the HRA form to complete at home, if desired. The form is returned when the employee returns to have the TB skin test evaluated. Allowing the employee to take the instrument home provides him or her with ample time to answer the questions thoughtfully.

Tying the return of the HRA to the TB test reading has increased the return rate of the completed form, thus assuring representation of a broader cross section of employees. The data is entered by staff at the Recreation Center of the health science center. The staff indicated their interest in collaboration in the health promotion and research efforts, and had the Wellsource computer program. Results are tabulated, and risk analysis is determined by the Wellsource program. The HRA's are scored and returned to UTNS-H within four days. The report is forwarded to the employee, accompanied by applicable health education information, influenced by the HRA findings. For example, if an employee is at risk for respiratory related disease due to anticipated occupational exposure and a past or current smoking history, information related to smoking cessation is included. When the self-reported diet history indicates high fat/low fiber intake, information about improving nutrition practices is made available. A letter is attached to the HRA summary, indicating pertinent points for the employee to note and helpful sources of referral within the health science center. In addition, health maintenance and screening information appropriate for age and gender is sent. Mammography, BSE, skin cancer, nutrition, exercise, and cholesterol information are included for all females; TSE and/or prostate cancer, skin cancer, nutrition, exercise, and cholesterol information are included for all males. If there is a particular high-risk problem identified in the HRA analysis, a personal phone call is made to the employee to elicit more information and plan appropriate follow-up.

RESEARCH STUDY USING HRA DATA

As Phase 1 of a longitudinal study to assess the long-term effectiveness of the use of HRA on the employee health program, analysis of the relationships among selected health indices were performed. Study of these relationships was initiated to answer the following questions:

1. What are the characteristics of employees who voluntarily participated in HRA in a worksite health program?
2. What are the relationships among demographics and risk indicators, for example, HRA subscores, in participants of the program?

Results of the analysis of the first year data indicate a relatively young sample with a mean age of 33.5. The group was approximately 67 percent female and 33 percent male. Most were educated at the college level, with approximately 17 percent having a master's degree or higher. This demographic profile is comparable to the population of new hires for the health science center in which 63 percent were female and 37 percent were male. The ethnic breakdown was predominantly Anglo (58 percent) with 24 percent African-American, 6 percent Hispanic, and 12 percent Asian. When comparing these percentages to all new hires, Anglos were represented proportionately, but African-Americans and Asians were overrepresented (24 percent compared to 19 percent and 12 percent compared to 10 percent, respectively) and Hispanics underrepresented (6 percent compared to 12 percent) in the study group. Approximately 9 percent were current smokers; 34 percent were over their recommended body weight. In the areas of heart health, stress/coping and safety employees were found to be functioning at a high to excellent wellness level; however, fitness, nutrition, and health practices scores fell in the low wellness area. A summary of HRA subscores for the total participant group is presented in Table 2.

For four aspects of wellness, a significant percentage of employees scored under the recommended level, indicating low levels of wellness. These included heart health (24 percent), stress/coping (38 percent), fitness (68 percent), and the number of health practices (73 percent). When gender comparisons were made, nonsignificant differences were found in most areas—number of health practices, nutrition, safety, or general wellness attitudes. Stress scores, however, indicated lower

Table 2   Characteristics of HRA subscores in employed workers.

Components of HRA	Mean	Rec*
Heart health	68	>60
Fitness	36	>60
Stress	85	>81
Nutrition	51	>60
Safety	43	>40
Health practices	4.8	> 6
Wellness attitude	58	>56
Overall wellness	64	>60

* Indicates the recommended scores based on normative data on which *Live Survey* analysis is based (Wellsource, 1989).

levels or perceived stress management for female participants, ($t = 2.39; p = .017$).

Discussion of Findings

It is important to note that this study utilized self-report data. Although the respondents were assured confidentiality, they may have been reluctant as newly hired employees in a predominantly health-oriented workplace to report less than optimal practices. The low prevalence of smoking, for example, may reflect this bias; also, the existence of a rebate for nonsmokers may have encouraged some employees to report nonsmoking behavior in all employment-related paperwork to assure this insurance incentive. Likewise, the positive attitudes toward wellness may be overreported. The very poor fitness and low average nutrition scores are sources of concern; if inflation of scores occurred due to response bias, the health status of the group may be even lower than indicated. Results of this descriptive survey certainly cannot be generalized to other working populations.

FINANCIAL ASPECTS

Evaluating the financial aspects of the HRA program brought to light some surprising figures. Table 3 provides the estimated costs of utilizing HRA's at UTNS-H during 1993. The estimated cost of $37.50 was incurred per HRA for each employee evaluated. This information on its own, however, does not answer the financial question. Two additional questions critical to this issue remain to be answered. (1) To what extent has long-term behavioral change resulted from the feedback to employees regarding their health risks after participation in the HRA? Some behavioral changes, smoking cessation or stress reduction, could be assumed to avert costly long-term illness. If cost-effectiveness were demonstrated quantitatively, administration may be willing to pay a higher reimbursement per employee in order to include health risk appraisal. (2) How does the individual employee perceive HRA to be beneficial to them? The employee may be willing to bear the additional cost in order to be given the HRA information. Preliminary data indicates that personnel costs within a university setting are prohibitively expensive for this particular program to be cost effective in its present form of implementation.

There are potential economic impacts of the use of HRA in a work setting, such as reduction in insurance claims, more

Table 3 Estimated costs of utilizing HRAs at UT Nursing Services—Houston.

Item	Cost per HRA ($)
Booklets	1.75
Office materials	1.17
Computer costs	8.65
Data entry person (salary & fringes)	1.50
Researcher/coordinator (salary & fringes)	15.63
LVN's/clerk (salary & fringes)	8.83
Total cost per HRA	37.50

appropriate utilization of health services, reduced absenteeism. An effective incentive that has not been widely investigated is insurance reimbursements when a follow-up HRA indicates positive behavioral changes in an employee's health habits. Since these aspects are not under the control of the nursing clinic, they were not explicitly evaluated. These areas need further exploration to evaluate financial implications for health promotion programs for the individual and the organization.

BENEFITS OF UTILIZING HRA AT UT NURSING SERVICES

The benefits of utilizing HRAs are many. First and foremost is the benefit to the participating new employees who were given an assessment of their health status and information regarding modifying identified health risks. In a follow-up survey conducted after one year, employees reported that they felt the process of participating in risk appraisal was valuable. Although the survey response rate was only 12 percent (51 out of a possible 418), 58 percent indicated that the HRA had been of above average or great benefit to them.

Second, as an educational institution, there is the expected emphasis on research. Gathering health risk data on over 400 new employees has created a significant database. This base of information serves as a foundation for the development of both individual and aggregate health education programs for the employees since a better appreciation of individual and aggregate health risks has been obtained. Further, this research database has served eleven master's degree students in the academic year 1992–1993 as sources of data for theses and research projects. Publications based on these data for both students and faculty will be the next logical outcome and are in progress.

Finally, the HRA is a marketing tool for the clinic. One of the target markets for primary care services includes employers of large organizations. Participants who indicated that the HRA was of benefit to them would be more likely to use the services of the clinic. The aggregate results of employee health risk appraisals can serve as feedback as to the overall health status of an employee. In turn, the employer can plan, develop, and deliver health education programs to meet the health care needs of the employees. Individuals who are apprised of their high risk status can use and do the nursing clinic for education, monitoring, and screening activities to modify their identified risks.

FUTURE UTILIZATION OF HRA AT UT NURSING SERVICES

This one year experience with HRA at UT Nursing Services-Houston has served as a lesson for future use of the instrument within the clinic. It has been an expensive, time-consuming, yet relatively high yielding information tool related to the health risks of the Health Science Center employees. There was a high level of perceived benefit reported from respondents to a follow-up survey. Further, this group reported that changes in their risk behaviors had occurred in response to the information on the health risk appraisal. Small to moderate changes in exercise were reported by 60 percent, while 65 percent stated that they had made nutritional modifications in the form of increasing fiber and decreasing fat in accordance with HRA recommendations. This project was not designed to measure clinical parameters, but changes in exercise and nutrition could be anticipated to result in improved health status and perhaps avoidance of disease. These long-term outcomes are in keeping with the goals of a nursing center.

A shorter version of the instrument is being considered for use. Retaining the benefit of participating in HRA in a more cost effective manner will be the desired outcome. Also, targeting the administration of the instrument to a specific department or group of employees rather than offering HRA to all new employees has been proposed. This would have the benefit

of economizing on staff and employee time needed to administer the HRA and could be followed with group instruction in
areas of greatest need for health education. Finally, the cost/
benefit of the use of HRAs in this population will continue to
be analyzed.

REFERENCES

AACN. (1992). *Special report on institutional resources and budgets in baccalaureate programs in nursing.*

Alexy, B. (1984). Health risk appraisal: Reliability demonstrated. *Proceedings of the society of prospective medicine,* (pp. 60–62). Indianapolis, IN.

Anderson, R., & Anderson, K. (1991). Worksite health promotion: The benefits of providing personal health status feedback and education programs to employees. *AAOHN Journal, 39*(2), 57–61.

Breslow, L., & Enstrom, J. (1980). Persistence of health habits and their relationship to mortality. *Preventive Medicine, 9,* 469–483.

Elias, W., & Dunton, S. (1980). Effect of reliability on risk factor estimation by a health hazard appraisal. *Proceedings of the 16th Annual Meeting of the Society of Prospective Medicine,* (pp. 1–5). Tucson, AZ.

Smith, K., McKinlay, S., & McKinlay, J. (1989). The reliability of health risk appraisals: A field trial of four instruments. *American Journal of Public Health, 79*(12), 1603–1607.

Smith, K., McKinlay, S., & McKinlay, J. (1991). The validity of health risk appraisals for coronary heart disease: Results from a randomized field trial. *American Journal of Public Health, 81*(4), 466–470.

Society of Prospective Medicine. (1992). *Directory of Health Risk Appraisals.* Indianapolis, IN.

Travis, J., & Callander, M. (1990). *Wellness for helping professions: Creating compassionate cultures.* Mill Valley, CA: Wellness Association Pub.

Warner, K., Wickizer, T., Wolfe, R., Schildroth, J., & Samuelson, M. (1988). Economic implications of workplace health promotion programs: Review of the literature. *Journal of Occupational Medicine, 30*(2), 106–112.

Wellsource Inc. (1989). *Life survey,* 2nd ed. Clakamas, OR.

Index

Academic nursing centers:
  faculty practice, 13
  financing, 11–12
  health care reform and,
    23–25
  liability insurance, 12
  mission, 12–13, 31
  organizational structure, 61
  research:
    directives for, 24
    studies of, 13–14
Access:
  expansion of, 15, 53
  research studies, 224–225
Accounting, business function
    modeling and, 63, 66
Accreditation, problems with, 9
Administration:
  APN role in, 18
  functions of, 10–11, 66
Adolescent care:
  adolescent, defined, 162
  advanced nurse practice, role
    in, 160–165
  at-risk adolescents, 170–173
  community agencies, 177
  need for, 177–178
  obstacles to, 162, 164
  rural health care clinics,
    173–177
  school health services, 165–170
  University of Rochester CNC,
    158–162
Adolescent specialists, role of, 174

Advance nurse practitioners
    (APNs), generally:
  physicians, competition with,
    7–8
  role in, 6–7
Advocacy, 41, 53
AIDS patients, care of, *see* Denver
    Nursing Project in Human
    Caring (DNPHC)/Caring
    Center
Alexy, B., 257, 265
Allen, K. D., 120, 133
Alpert, J. J., 185, 199
Ambulance services, 28
American Academy of Nurse
    Practitioners, 143
American Association of Colleges
    of Nursing (AACN), 100, 115,
    254, 265
American Journal of Nursing, 84, 96
American Nurses Association
    (ANA), 51, 55, 98, 100, 115,
    190, 200
American Public Health
    Association, 183, 200
Andersen, S., 231
Anderson, E., 155
Anderson, K., 255–256, 265
Anderson, R., 255–256, 265
Anderson, S., 133
Antonucci, T. C., 240, 251
Arizona Health Care Cost
    Containment System
    (AHCCCS), 182, 187, 197–199

Autonomous practice roles, 118
Autonomy, collaborative practice
   and, 29
Avorn, J., 118, 132, 146, 154
Aydelotte, M. K., 17, 216, 229

Bagwell, M. A., 218, 229
Baker, M., 118, 132, 146, 154
Bancroft, B., 164, 178
Barger, S., 17, 52, 55, 121, 132,
   217–218, 223, 229–230
Barkauska, V., 118, 133
Barrett, E. A. M., 43
Bauchner, H., 238, 251
Becker, E., 132
Bender, D. E., 103–104, 115
Berger, D. K., 191, 200
Berne, A. S., 236, 250
Bessman, A., 118, 132, 145, 154
Bibb, J., 164, 178
Billing systems, computerized,
   50–52
Biomore, T., 154
Birthing centers:
   accreditation of, 9
   financing, 11–12
   liability insurance and, 12
   Nursing Health Center model,
     91
Bless, C., 116
Blum, H. L., 185, 200
Boettcher, J. M. H., 218, 230
Branstetter, E., 17
Brodie, B., 164, 178
Breaking the Cycle of
   Disadvantage: A Nursing
   System of Health Care
   (Breaking the Cycle):
   funding, 183–184
   model:
     assessments, 188–189
     benefits of, 187–188
     medical supplies, 188

     personnel functions, 189–191
     services provided, 187
     staffing, 186–187
   planning and development,
     184
   purpose of, 181–182
Brecher, C., 32
Breslow, L., 257, 265
Bridgers, W. F., 216–217, 230
Bridges, W. C., 217–218, 230
Brown, S. A., 14, 17, 118, 132, 145,
   154
Brown, S. J., 241, 251
Browne, C., 118, 133
Brownlee, A., 116
Brownlee, S., 241–242, 251
Brykczynski, K. A., 241, 251
Budgeting, business function
   modeling and, 63, 66
Bulechek, G. M., 54–55
Business function modeling:
   defined, 62–63
   function/process groupings,
     64
   processes, 63–64, 120
Business planning:
   processes, 78–79
   software, 67–68
Business plans, 10

Call, R. L., 183, 200
Callander, M., 255, 265
Calmelat, A., 122, 132
Campbell, J., 118, 132
Capute, A. J., 242–243, 251
Caring center model, see Denver
   Department of Veterans
   Affairs Medical Center
   (DDVAMC), Caring Center
Carpentino, L., 54–55
Casamassimo, P. S., 183, 200
Centers for Disease Control, 256
Certificate of Need (CON), 91

DATE DUE

MAY 1 5 1996		
OCT 2 9 1996		
JAN 1 1 2002		